WEIGHT LOSS HYPNOSIS FOR WOMEN

A BLUEPRINT TO RAPID WEIGHT LOSS, FAT BURN, AND MOTIVATION THROUGH GASTRIC BAND HYPNOSIS, POSITIVE AFFIRMATIONS, AND GUIDED MEDITATIONS

J. W. CHLOE

SPECIAL BONUS!

Want This Bonus Book for **FREE**?

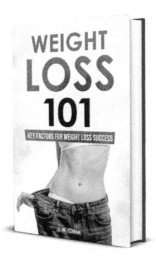

Get **FREE**, unlimited access to it and all my new books by joining the Fan Base!

***SCAN W/
YOUR PHONE
TO JOIN!***

CONTENTS

INTRODUCTION

Are you having trouble losing weight? Have you tried numerous options with little or no success? If this is you, then you are in the right place.

You will find this book useful if you are sick and tired of not fitting in the best pair of jeans, or if you are done counting calories and working out for countless hours. This book is also for individuals that have tried numerous solutions but haven't seen results yet. This book will help you to say goodbye to the extra pounds by discovering what works for you. You will learn here that weight loss doesn't have to be difficult regardless of your previous diets or workouts without results.

It is much easier than you can imagine! According to many globally respected institutions, hypnosis is effective for various medical ailments—including weight loss. This means that hypnosis could help you achieve your dream body without the stress of a complicated diet or regiment. For instance, you don't have to worry about counting calories with a food scale and converting them to Weight Watcher points.

Here is a sneak preview of what you will achieve after reading Weight Loss Hypnosis For Women – A Blueprint To Rapid Weight Loss, Fat Burn, and Motivation Through Gastric Band Hypnosis, Positive Affirmations, and Guided Meditations:

- You will develop a better and more positive view of your body.
- This book will also help you defeat cravings and binge eating naturally.
- You will also develop a healthier and more active lifestyle that will naturally help you avoid processed foods.
- Above all, you will end up loving yourself and your new lifestyle after realizing that you've found the perfect rhythm for maintaining a healthy lifestyle.

The book is divided into three key parts: Part one covers the theories of hypnosis. Feel free to skip this part and head straight to Part two if the first section isn't part of your weight loss journey. Part two is where the rubber meets the road. Here you will learn about the actual methods you will use to lose weight. Finally, part three is the icing on the cake. This part enlightens you on diets, nutrition, and how you can effectively track your weight loss progress.

Specifically, chapter one will help you understand hypnosis. You will also discover several hypnosis theories to help you understand the concept better. This will set the right foundation for the rest of the book.

In chapter two, you will learn how self-hypnosis can help you in your weight loss journey. Some of the details you will get in this chapter include how hypnosis works by targeting your subconscious mind. You will also learn how emotions affect your behavior and how you can use self-hypnosis to change undesirable behavior.

Chapter three meticulously covers the concept of gastric band therapy for weight loss. First, if you have never heard about it, I will let you in on what gastric band surgery is. After that, you will discover what gastric band hypnosis is and details on its success rate. I will also share some gastric band hypnosis scripts that you can use during your own journey.

Meditation for weight loss is another commonly miscon-strued concept. Chapter four will cover this subject in great detail and answer any questions you might be having. In this chapter, you will learn what meditation is and the different types of meditation to consider. I will also break down for you the use of mindful meditation as a weight loss tool. If you are a newbie to meditation for weight loss, you will also discover how you can start meditating, including guided imagery meditation and breathing techniques.

Chapter five will introduce you to the concept of positive affirmations for weight loss. First, we will thoroughly cover the law of attraction. Second, we'll discuss why having a healthy mindset matters in your weight loss journey. Third, we'll discover together what it means to love yourself and why you are worth it. Lastly, you will learn that weight loss is not a punishment. This chapter also explains how you can change your relationship with food and improve your emotional state. You will have access to several positive affirmations that you can use to get you started.

In chapter six, you will discover how you can create habits for weight loss. You will also learn about the difference between mindful and mindless eating. Since this book advocates for mindful eating, it will explain comprehensively how you can practice mindful eating. Some techniques you will learn include portion control, creating a routine, and setting up your home for success. You will also find out how to handle social situations in your weight loss journey.

Did you know that you need different kinds of motivation to keep you going in your weight loss journey? In chapter seven, I describe the subject of motivation for weight loss and share some best practices in detail. As you keep reading, you will learn about different kinds of inspiration and how you can create the right motivation for your weight loss journey. But, most importantly, this chapter will also teach you how to maintain sustainable motivation.

Many merchants who are out to fleece you to your last penny have misused dieting and eating principles. Even the Bible says, My people suffer for lack of knowledge. Thank God that you will not suffer for the same reason, for chapter eight will teach you the principles of dieting and eating right. With this knowledge, no one will be able to take advantage of your situation.

The chapter covers expansively why fad diets don't work and why you can use them and still fail to lose weight. It will also show you some different types of unsustainable diets that you should avoid. To better understand these principles, the chapter talks about eating disorders and weight stigma. It also discusses different factors that influence food choices and the role of the mind in weight loss. Lastly, you will equip yourself with the golden rules for eating and learn how to rewrite your brain for a healthy lifestyle.

Nutrition has principles that you must observe during your weight loss journey. Unfortunately, I have encountered many people who have used unhealthy methods that do not follow nutrition's unwavering principles to lose weight. As a result, their journey ended in tears. To avoid this predicament, I covered the principles of nutrition in chapter nine. Here you will read what proper nutrition means and how nutritional balance affects your weight loss success.

When you talk to any project manager, they will tell you monitoring and evaluation is a critical aspect of any project's success. In this regard, chapter ten will teach you how to track your progress during your weight loss journey. So what should you focus on? After reading this chapter, tracking your weight loss success will be more enjoyable than ever before. Remember, weight loss does not mean punishing your body.

In short, the contents of this book focuses on sustainability. The techniques covered in this book ensure that once you embark on your journey, you will not only enjoy it but also transform your life and achieve your goals. Above all, I want to ensure that you maintain your desired body weight as you enjoy your new lifestyle.

My background and personal experiences give me the confidence to share these things with you. I am a personal trainer, weight loss coach, and mindset coach. My line of duty has exposed me to numerous situations with different people so that I could help them with their weight loss struggles.

Besides my professional experience, I have also had my own struggles with body dysmorphic disorder and weight gain issues. After overcoming these issues, fitness and body recomposition became my life's passion. Nowadays, I find pleasure in helping people achieve success in their fitness and weight loss journey. In essence, it is what drives me each day! My interest in fitness has also enabled me to compete in bikini bodybuilding competitions on several occasions. However, I have retired from the competitive lifestyle, and retirement has allowed me to have more time to focus on helping others.

The knowledge I accumulated over the years has helped me successfully guide my clients throughout their weight loss journey. Many of them testify how my programs have helped them change their mindset on losing weight.

My passion for weight loss has also helped me learn everything I currently know about hypnosis and its significant effects on human body composition. I have also experimented with multiple hypnosis methods to discover precisely which one works best for weight loss. My motivation to write this book is to show you how easy and rewarding it is to use hypnosis methods to make long lasting changes to your stable weight. With these methods, you will inevitably lose weight, burn fat, and achieve your weight loss goals.

This book will not help you learn anything outside of the realm of weight loss hypnosis or weight loss in general. However, it is a guide that will teach you how to lose weight using different types of self-hypnosis techniques. In addition, it is an empowering book that will motivate you to make positive changes in your weight loss journey. As this book's title suggests, hypnosis is a great technique that has been scientifically proven to have positive results. It helps you reach inside and become a better version of yourself rather than just changing your appearance by losing weight.

Nevertheless, there is a lot of misunderstanding surrounding hypnosis that could make the title turn you away. So please bear with me and flip over to the first chapter so that you can understand the hypnosis I am talking about. It will be worth your while!

PART I

WHAT IS HYPNOSIS?

*H*ypnosis is a waking state of awareness in which your attention is detached from your immediate environment and is absorbed by your inner experiences like imagery, emotions, and cognition. Many people describe it as a sleep-like state, but you can express it better as a state of focused attention, increased suggestibility, and vivid fantasies. Even though people in a hypnotic state look like they are zoned out, in reality, they are usually in a state of hyper-awareness.

You will normally require the services of a certified hypnotist or hypnotherapist to guide you into a deep state of relaxation, also known as a trance-like state. Hypnotic induction entails focused attention and imaginative involvement until you reach the point when what you are imagining feels real. Once you get into this state, the hypnotherapist will give you suggestions designed to help you be more receptive to change or therapeutic improvement.

Beware of the many myths and misconceptions about hypnosis. For example, hypnosis is not therapy in itself. However, it is a very real process that can be used as a therapeutic tool. Hypnosis is used the same way a syringe is used to deliver drugs. It does not make the impossible possible, but it helps you believe and manifest what you can achieve.

Hypnosis has been used for medical and therapeutic purposes for a long time. It is predominantly used to reduce pain and anxiety among patients. The process has also proven helpful in helping individuals with behavioral disorders, such as eating disorders. For example, gastric band hypnotherapy has become a popular alternative for individuals considering gastric band surgery. It is less expensive, safer, and has recorded a success rate of over 90%.

THEORIES OF HYPNOSIS

For over 100 years, clinicians and scientists have proposed many theories to explain the phenomenon associated with hypnosis. The debate revolves mainly between state and non-state theories. Recent models of how the mind works, what is referred to as executive function, incorporate principles of cognitive psychology while current models utilize the concept of an Executive Control System (ECS). These two types of theories are differentiated by their properties, as shown in the table below:

State Theories	Non-State Theories
Hypnotic inductions create an altered state of consciousness.	Participants respond to suggestions nearly as well without hypnosis.
Hypnotic "trance" is associated with an altered state of brain function.	Participants in hypnosis experiments are actively engaged.
Responses to hypnotic suggestions are the result of special processes like dissociation or other altered states of consciousness.	Responses to suggestions are the product of normal psychological processes like expectancies, attitudes, and motivation.
Hypnotisability is extraordinarily stable over long periods.	Suggestibility can be modified using drugs or psychological processes.

State Theories

Hilgard's Neodissociation Theory (Hilgard, Crawford & Wert, 1979). Hilgard penned the neodissociation theory. This theory suggests that the hypnotic phenomenon is created through dissociation within a high-level, executive control system (ECS). In effect, Hilgard suggests that hypnotic induction splits the functioning of the ECS into distinct streams. Moreover, part of the ECS functions normally but cannot represent itself in conscious awareness because of the presence of an amnesic barrier.

According to Hilgard, hypnotic suggestions affect the disso-ciated part of the ECS. The subject is aware of the results of the suggestions but is not aware of the process by which they happen. He also claims that effective suggestions from the hypnotist take the majority of normal control from the subject. That means that the hypnotist will be able to influ-ence the executive functions and alter the structure of the target areas. When a subject is in a hypnotic state, their motor controls are altered, their memory and perception are distorted, and they perceive hallucinations as external reality.

Gruzelier's Neurophysiological Theory (Crawford & Gruzelier, 1992). The neurophysiological theory of hypnosis suggests that highly hypnotizable people have better executive function than hardly hypnotizable people and can separate their attention in different ways. In 1998, Gruzelier presented a model of hypnosis described by changes in brain function. The theory breaks down the process of hypnosis into three stages, each having its unique characteristics in brain activity patterns.

Gruzelier's neurophysiologic account suggests that changes to the attention control system's normal operations while in hypnosis are what make the subject more suggestible. During the first phase of the hypnotic induction, the subject pays close attention to the words of the hypnotist. There is increased activity in the left-sided, fronto-limbic brain regions.

In the second phase, the subject lets go of controlled attention and gives control to the hypnotist. There is reduced activity in the left frontal region during this phase. The subject engages in passive imagery in the third phase, displayed by the increased activity in the right-sided, temporo-posterior systems. Behavioral and neurophysiological evidence supports Gruzelier's theory. This theory also complements other state-like descriptions of hypnotic functioning.

Non-State Theories

Social-Cognitive Theory and Response Set Theory. According to the social-cognitive theory, the experience of effortlessness in hypnosis results from the subject's motivated predisposition to hypnotic suggestions because they do not require active planning and effort. In other words, effortlessness in hypnosis happens when subjects expect things to be effortless and choose to respond along with suggestions with no resistance. Implementation intentions are placed in the form: I will do y when x happens; while response expectancies are placed in the form: y will occur when x happens.

In 1997, Kirsch and Lynn suggested that subjects in a hypnotic situation have a generalized response expectancy. They will follow the instructions of the hypnotist and produce behaviors that feel involuntary. Consequently, subjects often attribute hypnotic responses to external causes and experience them involuntarily. This theory claims that hypnotic responses are initiated by the exact same mechanisms as voluntary responses. The only difference is how the subjects experience the behaviors.

Spanos's Socio-Cognitive Theory (Spanos & Chaves, 1989). This theory by Spanos and Chaves is also referred to as cognitive-behavioral perspective or social-psychological interpretation. According to Spanos, attitudes, imaginings, beliefs, expectancies, and attributions shape hypnotic phenomena. He used the construct of strategic role enactment to clarify how individuals transform thoughts, imaginings, and feelings into experiences and behaviors that are consistent with their thoughts of how a good hypnotic subject should respond to the overall hypnotic suggestions.

Spanos also opined that you could explain hypnotic behavior using the same social-psychological processes that explain non-hypnotic behaviors. He suggests that the active responses in hypnotizable people with analgesia and amnesia are not usually what they seem. According to Spanos, such responses reflect the normal social-cognitive processes.

Examples include compliance-induced biases, attentional focus alteration, and experience misattribution.

Kirsch's Response Expectancy Theory (Kirsch, 1985).

Kirsch came up with the response expectancy theory in 1985. He claimed that expectancies could directly alter an individual's subjective experience. When you expect a specific outcome, you sometimes subconsciously behave to produce that outcome.

Kirsch suggests that subjects in a hypnotic situation have a generalized response expectancy and that they will pursue the hypnotist's directives and generate behaviors that are still experienced involuntarily. Consequently, these subjects attribute hypnotic responses to external causes, which in this case is the hypnotist. This theory claims that hypnotic responses are initiated by the same mechanisms as voluntary responses, but the behaviors are experienced involuntarily.

Integrative Theories

Cold Control Theory (Dienes & Perner, 2007). The cold control theory of hypnosis reflects on the difference between control and awareness from the perspective of Rosenthal's Higher-Order Thought (HOT) theory. The HOT theory states that individuals are conscious of their mental states by having thoughts about those states. A thought about being in a mental state is a second-order thought (SOT) because it

is a mental state about a mental thought. It is also possible to have third-order thoughts when you become aware of having a SOT.

This theory claims that you can achieve a successful response to hypnotic suggestions by forming an intention to perform the action or cognitive activity required without forming the higher-order thoughts about intending that action that would usually accompany the performance of that action.

Brown & Oakley's Integrative Cognitive Theory (Brown & Oakley, 2004). Brown and Oakley emphasized the nature of perception and consciousness in this theory. They incorporated thoughts from the response set and dissociated control theories. They included the dissociated control theory suggestion that claimed responses could be facilitated by inhibition of high-level attention. Moreover, they included the response set idea that states that involuntariness is an attribution of behavioral causes.

Dissociated Control Theory (DCT) (Bowers, 1992; Woody & Bowers, 1994). The dissociated control theory of hypnosis uses the Norman and Shallice model of executive control to explain the hypnotic response. The initial model of the theory focused on a functional dissociation between executive control and the lower subsystem of control.

Woody & Bowers linked the theory to the Norman and Shallice concept formed in 1994.

The DCT model states that when highly hypnotizable individuals are hypnotized, the supervisory attentional system (SAS) becomes functionally dissociated from the contention scheduling system (CS). This means that the two levels stop working together.

The theory further states that when the higher-level control system is partly disabled, the subject becomes more dependent upon lower-level CS-based automatic processes. In effect, contextual cues and directions from the hypnotist affect the contention scheduling system and impact the experience of the hypnotized person.

Kihlstrom's Third Way (Kihlstrom, 2008). The third way theory of hypnosis is based on the notion that what we ought to do is clear, i.e. abandon the stand of either-or and adopt a new stance of both-and. This third way in hypnotic studies interprets hypnosis as both a state of profound cognitive change that involves basic mechanisms of cognition and consciousness and as a social interaction. Kihlstrom claims that the subject and the hypnotist come together for a particular purpose within a broad, social-cultural context.

KEY TAKEAWAYS

- Hypnosis is a highly misunderstood concept.
- There are rogue hypnotherapists. Before engaging with anyone you should ensure they have valid licenses and membership to one or more renowned associations.
- There are several theories that explain the concept of hypnosis.

Now that you have a clear understanding of what hypnosis is, you have a stronger foundation for understanding the other parts of this book. In the next chapter, you will learn how you can use self-hypnosis for weight loss.

HOW SELF-HYPNOSIS CAN AID IN WEIGHT LOSS

*Y*ou probably know about the typical go-to professionals like nutritionists, doctors, dietitians, and personal trainers that people seek out for weight loss matters. However, the thought of going to a hypnotist might not have crossed your mind. Nowadays, hypnosis is a well-known road used by many individuals who want to lose weight.

You see, healthy weight loss does not require a magic trick. Losing weight requires you to exercise regularly and make conscious choices about when, what, and how much to eat. Your progress depends on both your hormones and your health conditions. Your mind and emotions play critical roles in the weight loss journey, and this is where hypnotherapy and self-hypnosis become critical.

Hypnotherapy alone might not be sufficient to deliver dramatic weight loss results. However, sufficient evidence suggests that it can help subjects alter the beliefs and emotional connections they have that hamper their ability to modify their diet and exercise routines.

Two groups participated in a study in which they received individualized meal and exercise plans. One group also received training in how to use self-hypnosis techniques to boost their sense of self-control before eating. At the end of the trial period, the group that received self-hypnosis training had consumed fewer calories and had lost more weight on average. The self-hypnosis group also claimed that the quality of their life had improved.

It is also critical to note that the participants in the study worked with professional therapists to learn effective hypnotherapy techniques before attempting it on their own. Therefore, before practicing self-hypnosis, it is strongly recommended to attend at least one guided hypnotherapy session, led by a certified therapist, to learn the techniques.

Health professionals also claim that hypnotherapy is effective when it is combined with other weight loss measures. For instance, the experts suggest that hypnotherapy is most effective when combined with diet and exercise-based approaches.

HOW EXACTLY DOES SELF-HYPNOSIS FOR WEIGHT LOSS WORK?

Studies have investigated the effects of hypnotherapy on weight loss for several years. Below are the findings from that research.

It Helps Resolve Subconscious Emotional Conflicts

According to reports, hypnotherapy targets the unresolved emotional issues that hinder people from losing weight. For example, you can have all the information you need to lose weight, but you may still be eating for emotion rather than hunger. In such a case, you need to address the underlying emotions driving it.

This research reveals that an individual who experienced trauma, chaos, or abuse in the past may be unaware that their personal histories are affecting their current attempts to maintain a healthy weight. For such individuals, hypnotherapy can help heal the trauma, allowing the person to move on and release the weight.

It Helps Correct Errors in Thought Process and Negative Beliefs

Hypnosis also helps correct cultural misconceptions and faulty belief systems that limit an individual's ability to find a healthy weight. Experts point to the thin body ideals embedded in American culture as an example. Hypnotherapy can help by challenging a person's perception about how the human body should look. One health expert suggested that there is a misconception that thin bodies are healthy.

Moreover, people need to learn to appreciate changes in their bodies. For example, after childbirth or the natural aging process your, body will experience specific changes. If you appreciate these changes, it will help alleviate some of the stress and perfectionism that poisons weight loss goals.

Hypnosis can help the affected individuals correct some unhelpful beliefs, such as self-rewarding with food. For instance, instead of rewarding yourself with comfort food after a tough day, hypnosis can help you choose a reward that does not interfere with your healthy eating plans. You can learn to eat with a mindset of good health; hence going for treats that improve your health, which is actually what you deserve.

It Helps to Reduce Cravings

Hypnotherapy can help you reduce your desire for unhealthy foods. For instance, in an eat-well program, therapists use guided imagery and shared hypnotherapy sessions to lessen dietary cravings that could ruin your weight loss progress. Experts argue that once a subject is trained, they can use guided imagery and hypnotherapy to help themselves whenever they feel the need to.

SELF-HYPNOSIS FOR WEIGHT LOSS

Hypnotherapy sessions normally last between 50 minutes and 2 hours. The techniques might vary with the therapist you are using. However, many sessions begin with the subject finding a comfortable position, either lying down or seated.

Next, the therapist may ask you to close your eyes or focus on a specific object before leading you through a series of deep breathing exercises. As you begin to relax, the therapist will guide you to envision a safe and calming place like a body of water you love visiting. Once you enter a deeply relaxed state, also known as a trance, your therapist will suggest healthy thought patterns or beliefs to replace the ones you have that are not working in your favor.

Self-assuring words and phrases might also be part of your focus. Ultimately, your therapist will tenderly invite you to refocus your attention on the here and now. Once you master the process, you can use the meditative techniques independently with your needs. Some therapists will include a suggestion in your hypnosis session that will enable you to induce your own hypnotic state later.

FINAL THOUGHTS

Self-hypnosis is an effective way to lose some weight, especially when combined with diet and exercise modifications. The best way to get started is to work with a certified therapist who is specially trained for hypnotherapy. This will ensure that the techniques you learn will benefit you. Hypnotherapy can help you heal memories and emotions that disrupt your weight loss progress and is excellent for reinforcing healthy attitudes and correcting personal and cultural beliefs. The hypnotherapy will also help you reduce your desire for foods that you want to eliminate from your diet.

Remember, healthy weight loss is an individual process. Therefore, what works for your friends might not work for you. And what works in one period of your life might not be as effective in another. A supportive therapist that helps you relax and relearn habits through hypnotherapy will improve your odds of success.

KEY TAKEAWAYS

- There is no magic pill for weight loss.
- Hypnotherapy is a proven weight loss tool.
- You should seek the help of a professional hypnotherapist before you get started.
- You can effectively use self-hypnosis in your weight loss journey.

In the next chapter, you will learn about Gastric band hypnotherapy for weight loss.

PART II

GASTRIC BAND HYPNOTHERAPY FOR WEIGHT LOSS

*C*an hypnotic gastric banding help you lose weight? If that is your burning question, you have to read this chapter in its entirety. In matters of weight loss, you will be giving yourself false hope if you think there is a quick fix. Take a moment and think about the number of people struggling with overweight issues; it keeps increasing each year. Therefore, if we had a quick fix, we wouldn't be where we are today.

You have probably heard, read, or tried a few diet and exercise programs. However, individuals seem to be going for more drastic solutions to their weight problems now. Popular methods that have become trendy are gastric banding and gastric sleeve surgery. They both sound scary, don't they?

If you cannot afford the surgical procedure or are just afraid of going under the knife, you will be happy to hear there is a new solution in the weight loss scene. Have you ever heard of "virtual gastric banding" using hypnosis? If you are hearing this phrase for the first time, don't fret; you are in the right place. In this chapter, you will discover everything you need to know about gastric band hypnotherapy. You will first discover what a gastric band is and what the gastric band surgery entails. After that, you will be in a better position to understand gastric band hypnosis.

Does this new weight loss solution work? You will also find answers to that question in this chapter. Ultimately, you will be able to explain the gastric band hypnosis steps to anyone else in your life that may be interested as well.

WHAT IS THE GASTRIC BAND?

A gastric band is a device made of silicone that doctors use in a popular type of weight loss surgery. During the surgery, doctors place the band around the upper section of your stomach. The band helps create a small pouch of stomach above the device, restricting the amount of food that it can store. Afterward, it becomes difficult for you to eat large amounts.

The procedure is available through private surgery, and the major advantage of a gastric band is that it offers long-term, sustainable weight loss. However, you must strictly change your diet to experience the benefits of this procedure. In addition, you must exercise regularly and attend post-surgery appointments for any necessary support or advice.

The gastric band aims to restrict the amount of food you can physically consume. As a result, it causes you to feel full even after eating very little to speed up your weight loss. Gastric band surgery is usually the last resort for people who have unsuccessfully attempted other weight loss methods.

Like other surgical procedures, gastric band surgery has its risks. Here are some of the risks associated with having a physical gastric band:

- The band can slip out of place: When this happens, you could end up feeling sick, experiencing heartburn, or vomiting. You might have to undergo another surgical procedure to adjust or remove the band.
- Leaking in your gut: After a gastric bypass or gastric sleeve, different forms of the procedure, there is a small likelihood that food can leak into your abdomen. This leaking could cause a severe

infection, which could require antibiotics and surgery to repair the damage.

- Blocked Gut: Sometimes, the gastric band causes stomach blockages that induce vomiting, bowel issues, abdominal pain, and difficulty swallowing. This needs the attention of a professional surgeon to clear the blockages.

- Malnutrition: After the weight loss surgery, it might become difficult to absorb the right amount of vitamins and minerals. This means that affected individuals need to take supplements for the rest of their lives to avoid being malnourished.

Additionally, experts advise women who have had gastric band surgery to avoid getting pregnant for up to 18 months after the surgery. These risks must have scared you to death! But you can take it easy; hope is not gone. There is an alternative.

In the next part, we will cover the "virtual" gastric band or gastric band hypnosis.

WHAT EXACTLY IS GASTRIC BAND HYPNOSIS?

This is your go-to, weight loss method if you want to avoid the risks that come with the surgical procedure outlined in the previous section. It is also an ideal solution for individuals who do not qualify for the physical surgery. For gastric band hypnosis to work, the hypnotherapist uses a two-pronged approach.

First, they identify the root cause of your emotional eating. Experts describe emotional eating as a standard but unhealthy way of dealing with challenging feelings or emotions. For example, suppose you usually eat whenever you are stressed, or you use food to reward yourself after a tough week, or you eat when you are feeling bored. These are all signs of emotional eating.

With time, this behavior leads to feelings of shame, guilt, and sometimes a cycle of unhealthy eating habits. Eventually, you may even develop eating problems or physical health problems. A hypnotherapist uses hypnosis to help you remember the long-forgotten experiences surrounding food that could be affecting your diet without your knowledge. The hypnosis process will also help you recognize reactions, patterns, and behaviors that you might not realize you are doing. It is essential to identify and address unhealthy thought patterns surrounding food before beginning gastric band hypnotherapy.

Second, the hypnotherapist will carry out the virtual gastric treatment. Gastric band hypnotherapy works by suggesting that you have had an operation that inserts a small gastric band but at a subconscious level. The procedure's objective is for your body to respond to this proposition by making you feel full quicker as though you had the actual surgery. Think of it as a placebo.

Getting a virtual gastric band is different from fad diets, as the therapists have designed it to help you make beneficial, lifestyle changes. Hypnotherapy helps you to take the first steps towards positive living by:

- Helping you recognize and address any underlying issues.
- Helping you identify food-related triggers.
- Working with your subconscious to help you feel fuller for a longer period.

One hypnotherapist argued that diets don't usually deal with the necessary, permanent lifestyle changes like sustainable, long-term changes in a person's eating habits and food attitudes. According to the experts, several diet plans offer temporary solutions. However, they are usually challenging to maintain because they can be too restrictive or totally deprive you of your favorite foods. In addition, most diet plans tend to make you more obsessed with food as eating requires counting calories and consciously measuring portion sizes.

HOW GASTRIC BAND HYPNOSIS WORKS

A hypnotherapist will use relaxation techniques to put you into a state of hypnosis. While you are in a relaxed state, your subconscious becomes more open to the suggestions to come. It is at this point that your hypnotherapist will make suggestions to your subconscious. For example, during a gastric band hypnotherapy session, the hypnotherapist will suggest that he has fitted you with a physical band.

Your mind is more powerful than you imagine. If your subconscious believes in these suggestions, then your behavior changes accordingly. Typically, the therapist will also include other suggestions surrounding confidence and behavior to help you commit to the changes in lifestyle. Many therapists will also teach you self-hypnosis techniques that you can do at home to help you enhance the work you have accomplished after the session is over. You are also advised to enlighten yourself on nutrition and physical exercise to strengthen your physical health and well-being.

DO YOU HAVE UNHEALTHY RELATIONSHIPS WITH FOOD?

Changing your relationship with food is essential for gastric band hypnotherapy to work. If you simply focus on the end goal of losing weight, you are likely going to overlook fundamental issues, like having an unhealthy relationship with food. These underlying issues with food could also be affecting other areas in your life, causing feelings of anxiety, guilt, and sometimes hindering you in social situations.

What should you expect when getting a virtual gastric band?

By now, you already know that the hypnotherapist will not cut you open. So if you are not a friend of the surgical blades, you are safe. In this part, you will discover the things you will encounter during the therapy sessions.

In your first meeting with your hypnotherapist, you will discuss your objectives. This is a chance for you to open up about your previous attempts to lose weight, eating habits, health issues, and your overall attitude towards food. If you have any health issues relating to your weight, please seek advice from your doctor. This information will help the hypnotherapist understand what will be beneficial to your case. It will also help the hypnotherapist determine whether you will require other forms of treatment.

The gastric band hypnosis procedure is designed to imitate the actual gastric band surgery to help your subconscious think that it really happened. Many hypnotherapists usually incorporate the smells and sounds of an operating theatre to make the experience more authentic. The therapist will start by guiding you into a deeply relaxed state, also known as hypnosis. You will be aware of the goings-on and will be in control at all times. So don't worry about the misconceptions about being peddled during hypnotherapy sessions.

The moment you are in the hypnotic state, your hypnotherapist will talk you through the "operation." They usually explain bit by bit what happens in surgery, including being put under the anesthetic, the first incision, fitting the band, and stitching up the incision. The sounds and smells of an authentic operating theatre will boost the experience, persuading your subconscious that whatever the therapist is saying is actually happening to you.

Your hypnotherapist might include other suggestions during the session to boost your self-confidence. After the procedure is complete, your therapist may teach you some additional self-hypnosis techniques to help you stay on track. Some hypnotherapists may request you to return for follow-up appointments so they can observe the virtual gastric band's effectiveness and make any necessary adjustments.

It is important to note that individuals with a physical gastric band also benefit from these hypnotherapy sessions. The sessions will help the subject address underlying issues surrounding self-esteem and food. You should also use gastric band hypnosis alongside other weight-management methods that deal with exercise habits and nutrition. An effective weight loss program must blend body and mind-changing habits.

ARE YOU READY TO GO FOR VIRTUAL GASTRIC BAND HYPNOTHERAPY?

If your answer is yes, that is great! However, there are certain things you need to consider while selecting your hypnotherapist. The industry is mostly unregulated, meaning that anyone can masquerade as a hypnotherapist. In this regard, you should know what to look for before booking an appointment with a hypnotherapist.

According to reputable industry experts, here is what to look for:

- Your hypnotherapist must be a member of a reputable hypnotherapy association. The associations usually supervise and train their members regularly. Moreover, they also ensure that the hypnotherapists have minimum requirements of job experience and training.
- The therapists should also have accreditation from a hypnotherapy association. Some of the

associations accredit members based on their studies and experience.

- It will be best to work with a practitioner that has a first aid qualification. They should also have completed a background check and have public indemnity insurance.
- The experts also advise that you should go for a hypnotherapist that has other skills like counseling. Some are registered psychologists who employ hypnotherapy as one of their techniques.
- It is also wise to speak with the hypnotherapist before you make an appointment for a paid consultation. This step allows you to verify their qualifications and get a sense of their personality to make sure your personalities match.
- You are also advised to be price aware. Even though the practitioners follow no set pricing model, experts recommend not paying more than 250 USD.
- Remember to consider the number of sessions. The number of hypnotherapy sessions you require depends on what you are being treated for. Nevertheless, experts warn that you should look for someone else if you don't feel any connection with your therapist during the first session.

VIRTUAL GASTRIC BAND HYPNOSIS SHOULD BE TAILORED TO AN INDIVIDUAL

According to experts, for this program to succeed, it needs to be customized to your individual needs. Virtual gastric band hypnosis works by providing emotional healing and enabling you to reach your weight loss goals. Apart from eliminating food cravings, it also helps to remove negative emotions related to certain memories.

The suggestions have to be explicitly tailored to your unique situation and outlook for it to work. This means that virtual gastric band hypnotherapy does not have a one-size-fits-all solution. If you go to a therapist who seems to be reading from a script, your chances of success are minimal.

WHAT IS THE SUCCESS RATE OF THIS METHOD?

Clinical research has revealed that there is a 95% success rate for virtual gastric band hypnosis programs in the United Kingdom. However, the study also stated that the remaining 5% were unsuccessful because they were highly closed to the therapy session. Moreover, the subjects were unable to relax enough for the therapist's words to have any real effect.

Other reports suggest that the therapy begins working after the first session. However, if it does not work, the therapist might schedule other sessions until the results are satisfactory. Patients who gave up after the first session and never returned were also counted as part of that 5%. Hypnotherapy is not for everyone. The program only works for individuals who are ready to change their feelings toward food. If you don't want it to work, you won't do anything that will earn you satisfactory results.

GASTRIC BAND HYPNOSIS METHOD AND STEPS WITH SCRIPT EXAMPLES

Here is an extract from a virtual gastric band (phase 1) script:

"And here we are.

Please make yourself comfortable . . . settle in . . . and don't worry about how deeply you have to relax to enter into a trance . . . you don't even have to try. In fact, trying too hard to relax may prevent you from going deeper into yourself, where your unconscious mind is waiting for answers that will heal you.

So . . . just listen, as there are important reasons why you're here today, aren't there?

And take a deep breath . . . and another . . . and continue to notice your slow and steady breathing, paying close attention to the feeling of your chest rising and falling. Allowing it to rise . . . almost on its own . . . and feel that positive air pressure with the incoming breath and, as you release the air, letting it slowly escape on it's own notice that your chest is relaxing and releasing pressure as the air escapes.

You can even imagine the air being a certain, healing color as it enters and leaves your body, leading you further into a deeply relaxed state. Not because you're forcing it to happen. Because deep relaxation happens all by itself, does it not? When you allow it to happen . . . when you give into the relaxation and ease of simply being where you are right now.

As you continue to enjoy a state of relaxation, you become aware of your desire to lose weight. You may have been seeking solutions for some time. You're tired and frustrated with yourself . . . with how difficult it's been . . . You may not have even believed it possible to lose weight. Still, there's a strong desire within you to be healthy, fit, and comfortable in your body. You want to lose weight, and it's time to heal the part of you that doesn't want you to lose that weight.

That's right . . . the part of you that doesn't want to lose weight . . . that may even want, or insist, on sabotaging your efforts to be healthy. This is a powerful part of you that you've been wishing to simply go away and leave you in peace.

Yet, this part of you doesn't listen, does it? It has a mind of its own. It's your own agenda that you now have the opportunity to reconcile within yourself so that you can move on . . . slowly, steadily, and successfully arriving at your ideal weight.

And that part of you may be rebelling against your goal, right? Even if you're not aware right now of seeing, hearing, or feeling something on the inside that represents the rebellion. That protest . . . that part of you who insists on sabotaging your weight loss will show up. Maybe late at night, maybe in a moment of weakness, or laziness, or temptation, or self-indulgence. This inner weight loss saboteur is lurking in the background, waiting to strike.

And you can face that part of you now . . . not as an enemy . . . not as a victim . . . but as a long, lost friend. This part of you is the part that is hurt, outcast and rejected by others . . . rejected by you, and now is the time to heal. Isn't it time to extend a healing hand to yourself. Is now not the moment to make peace with yourself?

Allow this to happen. You can say to this part of you what you've always wanted to hear. Allow those words to sink in as you hear them: I'm sorry you're hurt. You've been hurt by others. You've been ignored by me. I've wished you would just disappear, and now I know that's not fair to you. It's time to heal . . . and I'd like you to feel loved . . . included in my life. I'd like to be here for you and ask that you support me as well. Let's work together. Let's end this war. We can make peace. It's up to us and no one else, isn't it?

Imagine making peace with yourself, right now, and feeling a healing energy pass through your body that touches all parts of you . . . bringing together your strengths and resources, healing your weaknesses and bridging the divide that's been in your soul . . . keeping you from wholly embracing your healthiest sense of self.

You get to be a whole person. A genuine and integrated human being, with all your strengths accessible to all parts of yourself.

And you can feel proud of yourself and motivated by your courage to face yourself and begin a healing process that doesn't end with this session, but continues on its own, showing up in your thoughts and feelings . . . and your dreams . . . with even more healing benefits that may surprise you.

And you'll soon discover all parts of yourself aligning toward your healthiest sense of self . . . physically, mentally, emotionally, and spiritually. Healthy food will taste wonderful. Unhealthy food will taste fake and empty and lifeless. You'll be motivated to move your body and invite a vibrant feeling of overall well-being and fitness. And when you feel the temptation to go off course, to sabotage your weight loss, you'll feel an immediate sense of compassion for yourself, make peace on the inside, and remain strong on the outside.

Weight loss, in this way, will come naturally.

Now . . . take your time . . . allow what you've learned in this session to integrate into your being . . . and when you choose to return your attention to the room you're in, you'll feel relaxed, awake, and full of hope."

CASE STUDY: ONE-SIZE-FITS-ALL DOES NOT WORK IN VIRTUAL GASTRIC BAND HYPNOTHERAPY

Lucy from Maryland says the concept of virtual gastric banding appealed to her because it seemed like a less severe alternative to the real gastric banding procedure. She revealed that she has been grappling with her weight and has still been gaining weight for a while. She had tried all options with no success and was considering going for a gastric lap band surgery.

During her research, she came across websites offering the hypnosis version and decided it was worth a try. Lucy got in touch with a hypnotherapist in her local area who claimed to do virtual gastric banding and made an appointment. However, she admits she did not know what to look for when choosing a hypnotherapist. So she did not think to check the therapist's qualifications before booking her first session, which cost 200 USD.

During the session, the therapist made her sit in a comfortable chair with a blanket. He then started the process of putting her under by speaking while a soundtrack of beeping and other operating theater noises played in the background.

Lucy, a nurse, had difficulty entering a relaxed state as there was something off with the hospital soundtrack. She described what it was like to lay there thinking that it was not the correct machine or noise, which made it hard for her to go under. She also stated that the therapist appeared to be reading from a script that gave the entire session a generic feel. Lucy was also shocked that the therapist did not talk to her about anything before the session. He did not ask her about her weight loss issues, her job, or her regular habits.

After the session, he gave Lucy a CD with a follow-up soundtrack to listen to when she got home. He also asked her to come back for more sessions. And you guessed it!

Lucy never went back for another session because the first one felt like a total waste of her money and time.

Lucy was disappointed that the hypnotherapist did not even try to customize his approach to suit her unique needs. She came to the conclusion that the gastric banding approach wasn't working, she expected the therapist to try something different. But, instead, it just felt like a one-size-fits-all process!

KEY TAKEAWAYS

- Virtual gastric banding is a practical alternative to real gastric band surgery.
- Gastric band hypnosis works well when integrated with other nutrition and physical exercise programs.
- Not all subjects are eligible for gastric band hypnosis.
- You should confirm the qualifications of your therapist before booking an appointment.
- One size does not fit all when it comes to gastric band hypnotherapy sessions. You should find a practitioner that can tailor the therapy session to your specific needs.

BOTTOM LINE

If you have tried gastric band hypnosis and have failed, don't despair. There are still many other alternatives that you can pursue to help you shed weight. In the next chapter, we'll discuss how you can use meditation to lose weight.

4

MEDITATION FOR WEIGHT LOSS

*S*uppose your ideas for weight loss are only accurate to some extent. Have you ever wondered if there is more at stake than changing your diet and physical exercise? A friend of mine discovered something new when she signed up for a modeling contract at 16 years old. Her agents immediately told her that she would have to "stay skinny" and "refrain from eating a lot until next week."

Because of the pressure that came with trying to stay skinny, things became complicated over the next ten years of her life; she revealed how she developed a fear and anxiety around weight that consumed her life. The condition got worse when she woke up in a hospital bed with anorexia so severe that it nearly killed her. The emergency room staff advised her that she needed to make adjustments to her lifestyle if she wanted to live, and it is at this point that she discovered her saving grace—meditation.

If you are like my friend, today is your lucky day. In this chapter, I will cover everything you need to know about meditation in-depth. First, you will learn what meditation is and then we'll uncover the different types of meditation. After that, we'll talk about how meditation affects weight loss and how to start meditating today. Finally, towards the end of the chapter, there will be guided meditation scripts and steps.

WHAT IS MEDITATION

Meditation is a daily exercise that requires you to clear your mind and return to a place where your thinking is straightforward and your emotions are calm. Experts suggest that a good meditation session should last for at least 20 minutes and be repeated every day.

Contrary to popular belief, meditation does not have to be complicated. If you are still new to this habit, you can start by taking five minutes immediately after you wake up to clear your mind before you embark on your daily activities. Then close your eyes and focus on your breathing pattern without trying to change it. At first, your mind will likely wander, and if that happens, gently guide it back to your breathing.

Even though experts suggest that you should practice meditation for at least 20 minutes every day (10 minutes in the morning and 10 in the evening), it is essential to note that the amount of time you spend meditating is not as important as how regularly you do it. Of course, it is usually challenging to form new habits, so start with five-minute meditation sessions every day.

HOW TO MEDITATE

There are several ways to meditate. Nevertheless, most meditation types follow a specific pattern that has these four things:

1. **A serene location:** It is up to you to choose where to meditate. It could be your favorite chair, lying down on your bed, or while on a walk.
2. **A specific, relaxed posture:** For example, you may feel most relaxed when you are sitting, walking, standing, or lying down.
3. **Focused attention:** You can choose to focus on your breath, a word, a phrase, or anything else.
4. **An open attitude:** It is typical to have other

thoughts while meditating, but try not to focus on these thoughts. Keep directing your focus back to your breath, or whatever else you chose to focus on.

If you are just starting, it will help to take a class to learn the basics of meditation.

DON'T JUDGE, BE A WITNESS!

Meditation requires you to commit and stop to look within and around you, even if it is for a few minutes. Meditation experts argue that your focus should be on witnessing your thoughts instead of focusing on how long you need to meditate. The aim is to learn how to quiet your mind and, at times, steer clear of the false or stressful stories you usually tell yourself.

It would be helpful if you did not bring any major expectations to meditation. Just let it unfold devoid of judgment. Many people carry around an inner critic who runs their lives. Because of this, experts suggest that you reframe your thinking by asking, what's working? whenever you wake up and again at the end of your busy day.

People often get so caught up in their daily hustle and bustle that they do not take the time to find out and appreciate what is good. Instead, experts suggest that people need to take a moment and look around to recognize what is in front of them. It is one of the many ways to be present. However, you do not need to be present just in the moment but also informed to make the right decisions. For example, be aware of your lifestyle choices regarding what to eat and what you should avoid—and the best exercises to lose weight.

In short, meditation does not replace other weight loss activities such as diet and exercise. Instead, it supports the positive changes that come with those things as long as you are patient and committed. You are now ready to discover the different types of meditation.

THE DIFFERENT TYPES OF MEDITATION

There are many different types of meditation. However, this section will focus on the nine main types of meditation. It is important to remember that there is no right or wrong way to meditate. However, make sure you find a practice that caters to your needs and works well with your personality.

Meditation experts warn that not all meditation styles are suitable for you. Different meditation styles each require specific skills and mindsets. So you might be asking: How do I know which practice is best for me? Well, simply go for whatever feels comfortable.

Here are the main types of meditation:

Mindfulness Meditation

This kind of meditation has its roots in Buddhist teachings. It is also regarded as the most popular meditation technique in Western countries. In mindfulness meditation, the subject focuses on their thoughts as each one passes through their mind. During the process, you don't judge or get involved in the thoughts; you just observe and note any patterns.

This exercise integrates concentration and awareness. It will help you to focus on a particular thing, like your breath or an object, as you observe any bodily sensations, feelings, or thoughts. Mindfulness meditation is best suited for individuals who don't have a teacher to guide them because you can effortlessly practice it alone.

Spiritual Meditation

Spiritual Meditation is prevalent in Eastern religions like Daoism, Hinduism, and also in some Christian practices. It works like a prayer where you reflect on the silence around you as you look for a deeper connection with God or the Universe. Many people use essential oils to heighten the spiritual experience. Commonly used scents include palo santo, cedar, sage, frankincense, and myrrh.

You can do spiritual meditation at home or in a place of worship. This type of meditation is for individuals who thrive in silence and are interested in spiritual growth as well.

Focused Meditation

Focused meditation entails concentration using any of the five senses. For instance, you can choose to focus on an internal thing like your breath, or you can bring in external influences to help focus your attention. For example, you can count mala beads, listen to the strike of a gong, or stare at a candle flame. This kind of meditation sounds simple in theory, but can be a bit challenging for beginners to hold their focus for more than a few minutes.

Whenever your mind wanders, it is critical to bring it back to the subject of attention. This kind of meditation is for individuals that need additional focus in their lives.

Movement Meditation

What comes to mind when you hear movement meditation? Of course you are thinking of yoga. However, there is more than just that! Movement meditation can also be walking through the woods, tai chi, gardening, or any other gentle form of movement.

It is an active kind of meditation that uses movement to guide the subject. This type of meditation works for people who find peace in action and prefer their minds to wander.

Mantra Meditation

Mantra meditation is prevalent in many teachings, for example, Buddhist and Hindu traditions. This type of meditation utilizes repetitive sound to help clear the mind. The repetitive sound can be a phrase or word like the famous "om" associated with meditating.

It does not matter whether you vocalize the mantra loudly or quietly. Once you chant your mantra for a while, you become more alert and connected to your environment. This state allows you to experience deeper levels of awareness.

If it is easier for you to focus on a word than your breath, you will enjoy mantra meditation more. It is also the go-to meditation type if silence does not work for you and repetition clears your mind.

Transcendental Meditation

Transcendental meditation is a famous type of meditation. It is featured predominantly in several studies in the scientific community. This type of meditation is more customizable than mantra meditation. It uses a mantra or a series of words specific to each practitioner.

Individuals who like structure and can commit to maintaining a regular practice find the most benefits from this type of meditation.

Progressive Relaxation

Progressive relaxation is also known as scan meditation. It is a practice that aims to reduce tension in your body with the goal being to promote relaxation. Usually, this type of meditation involves gradually tightening and relaxing one muscle group at a time throughout your body.

In some instances, a guide might encourage the subject to imagine a gentle wave flowing through their body to help release any pressure. It is an ideal form of meditation for relieving stress and unwinding before you go to bed.

Loving-Kindness Meditation

This kind of meditation builds up feelings of compassion, kindness, and acceptance towards yourself and others. It usually involves opening your mind to receive love from others and then taking time to send several well wishes to friends, acquaintances, and loved ones.

This is a perfect form of meditation for individuals struggling with resentment or feelings of anger because it promotes the development of regular kindness and compassion.

Visualization Meditation

Visualization meditation is a practice that aims to promote the feelings of peace, relaxation, and calmness through visualizing positive images and scenes. With this type of meditation, it is essential to imagine the scene vividly and use all five senses to include as much detail possible.

There is another form of visualization meditation that involves imagining yourself succeeding at specific goals. This type of meditation aims to increase your focus and motivation. Most people use this kind of meditation to boost their mood, promote inner peace, and reduce stress levels.

HOW MEDITATION AFFECTS WEIGHT LOSS – MINDFUL MEDITATION AS A TOOL FOR WEIGHT LOSS

What is the connection between meditation and weight loss? According to research findings, meditation is an effective tool that helps individuals lose weight. The studies suggest that meditation is powerful because it aligns the conscious and unconscious mind to agree on the behavioral changes you want to make. Examples of behavioral changes you may want to make include controlling cravings for unhealthy food and changing your overall eating habits.

Your unconscious mind must be involved because that is where detrimental, weight-gaining behavior like emotional eating is deeply rooted. Meditation will help you become more aware of these issues, override them with practice, and replace them with slimming habits.

Meditation experts also argue that this method has more immediate effects. For instance, it will help you reduce levels of stress hormones, like cortisol, that signal your body to store calories as visceral fat. You see, if you have a lot of cortisol pumping through your body, it will be difficult to shed weight even if you are making the right choices.

That sounds complicated, right? It's not uncommon for people to be stressed, and it is usually not that simple to shake the stress off. However, it only takes about 25 minutes of meditation for 3 consecutive days to significantly reduce your stress levels.

HOW MEDITATION HELPS YOU MANAGE YOUR WEIGHT

When you think about losing weight, you are likely to go for the obvious solutions like participating in a spin class or going for a salad instead of a sumptuous burger. Consequently, you might consider it nonsensical to sit in a single place and focus on your thoughts, meditating for weight loss. This mindset has a limited view of what weight loss involves. Remember, weight loss is not just a physical thing, and human beings are also emotional beings. If you can use this to your advantage, it will go a long way in helping you develop a healthy relationship with food. As a result, you will shed body fat or, at least, maintain the weight that is healthiest for your body.

Studies on this subject have found that typical weight loss methods, including exercise and diet, only work in the short-term. Research also shows that the individuals who took part in the study usually gained their weight back after the program ended. On the flip side, the weight loss protocols that incorporated mindfulness interventions, like meditation, were seen to be more effective in weight loss and maintaining body shape. So how does meditation help you lose weight?

Meditation works physically and psychologically. For example, meditation helps reduce the levels of cortisol and C-reactive protein in your physical body. And psychological studies have confirmed that meditation can also help get rid of overeating.

How Meditation Helps You Create a Healthy Relationship With Eating

Meditation helps the participants to become more mindful eaters. It also helps them address any emotional eating issues that persist. Here is how meditation helps:

- **By removing shame and guilt:** If you struggle with emotional eating when you feel stressed, you could end up overeating to relieve some of that feeling of stress. This usually leads to guilt or shame. Meditation will help you to reduce the stress levels, which attacks the trigger of the problem. It also allows you to be more aware of your feelings and emotions, enabling you to differentiate when you are eating because of stress and when you are hungry.

- **By maintaining your weight loss in the long-term:** Meditation can help you maintain your weight loss progress. Diet and exercise will enable you to reach your goals. But it's meditation, exercise, and healthy eating that will help you sustain your weight loss efforts.

- **By lowering stress and inflammation levels:** As mentioned earlier, meditation helps to reduce someone's C-reactive and cortisol levels.

This is excellent for your overall health and will aid in achieving your weight loss objectives.

- **By giving you better control of your cravings:** People who are struggling with emotional eating find it difficult to manage intense cravings. According to studies, mindfulness meditation can help you address this hard-to-control behavior.
- **By reducing stress and anxiety:** The weight loss journey can be stressful, leading to an increase in anxiety. Daily meditation will help you reduce, and be aware, of your anxiety levels.

HOW TO START MEDITATING

If you have a mind and body, you can practice meditation. You don't need special equipment or expensive classes to get started. For many individuals, the most challenging part is finding the time. The best approach is to start off with something reasonable—like 10 minutes every day.

Before you get started, please ensure you have a quiet place that you can use for 10 minutes. Here are some tips to get started:

- Get rid of the distractions, including screens when you are eating. For instance, switch off the television, put your phone away, and step away from your computer table.

- Eat slowly and chew your food thoroughly. Try to make a check-in halfway through your meal to evaluate how you are feeling. An essential thing you should be asking yourself is whether you are still hungry or are beginning to feel full.

- Write down your senses. Ensure your senses are part of your mindful-eating program. Focus on your food's smell, taste, and flavors. You should also try to note the various textures.

- How do you feel as you eat the food? Do you feel sleepy? Energized? Do you experience an upset stomach or bloating afterward? Did the meal keep you full or were you hungry almost immediately?

- Don't judge yourself harshly. Mindful eating can be complex, and it takes time to learn how to do it effectively. Don't beat yourself up if you mess up or forget. Relaxing is part of the process.

- Stay in touch with your feelings. Why are you eating? Is it because you are feeling hungry, or is there an emotion behind your craving?

Now that you've read through these tips, you are ready to get started. First, go to your quiet place and make yourself comfortable. You are free to lie down or sit in any position that makes you feel relaxed.

After that, shift your focus to your breathing and watch your stomach or chest as it falls and rises. Try to feel the air as it moves in and out of your nose or mouth. Listen to the sounds the air makes as you breathe. Do this for up to 2 minutes or until you start feeling thoroughly relaxed.

With your eyes opened or closed, follow these steps:

1. Breathe in deeply and hold it for several seconds.
2. Exhale slowly and repeat.
3. Breathe naturally.
4. Examine your breath as it goes through your nostrils, raising your chest and moving your belly. Please don't force your breathing in any way.
5. For the next 5 to 10 minutes, keep focusing on your breath.
6. Your mind will start wandering. Don't worry; it is normal. Simply acknowledge that your mind has gone off track and return your focus to your breaths.
7. As you start to wrap up, reflect on how it was easy for your mind to wander. After that, acknowledge how it was easy for you to bring your attention back to your breathing.

Try to do this exercise as many days each week as you can. Remember, it might not feel effective in the first few sessions. However, with regular practice, it will become easier and will start feeling more natural. You can also find phone apps and YouTube videos that can guide you through mindfulness meditation.

GUIDED MEDITATION SCRIPTS AND STEPS – LAYOUT THE PROCEDURE

Below you will find a guided meditation script that will help you see yourself as the person you wish to be. The meditation is gentle and empowering, and you can apply it as an everyday tool to help you lose weight.

A Meditation for Weight Loss

"Welcome

If you are using this meditation, please remember that you should want to lose weight for yourself or for health reasons, not because of external pressures that claim you have to be thin to be accepted.

You are already a wonderful and unique person, and we want you to keep that in mind throughout this meditation and every moment of every day following.

This short mediation is all about changing your perception of yourself and should be practiced each day until you can easily see the you that you wish to be.

Find a quiet place where you will not be disturbed for a few minutes. You may also practice this meditation before you go to sleep. Close your eyes and breathe slowly in through your nose and out through your mouth, letting your breathing fall into a natural rhythm.

If other thoughts enter your mind, don't interact with them. Simply watch them come and watch them go like clouds across the sky and return your focus to your breath.

Imagine yourself sitting in a beautiful garden. There is a small green lawn and banks of flowers around you surrounded by trees. You see someone walking towards you from the end of the garden. They are smiling . . . They look incredibly happy . . . That person is you—you as you wish to be.

They are wearing something you would love to wear. They are just the size you would want to be, and they are glowing with health and vitality. Their eyes are brilliant and clear, and you can feel the excitement and pleasure of you looking and feeling so amazing.

Admire yourself wholeheartedly.

Imagine yourself in different outfits wearing each one with complete confidence and looking absolutely wonderful. Remember this image of yourself whenever you look in the mirror. Whenever you think of yourself, bring to mind the person you saw inside this meditation.

The more you do this, the easier and more automatic it will become. The person you want to become is already there; you are becoming that person every second, minute, and hour night and day.

Already you are beautiful, incredible, and amazing, and you must recognize that. The new you is actually you, not a different person; not an unattainable goal or dream.

That person is you."

MEDITATION FOR WEIGHT LOSS: CASE STUDY

Subject: Chloe Mathison

Age: 40

Height: 5'4"

Beginning weight: 297 lbs.

How She Gained Weight:

Her childhood was filled with food-related memories. She used to help her parents in the back of their restaurant. On top of that, she would also have a full breakfast with her dad every morning before going to school. She even used to make several trips to buy candy bars for her mum throughout the week.

By the time she was in her early 20s, she was weighing in at 225 pounds. Several years later, she got married, and her weight kept increasing as she spiraled into depression. She was a teacher and had developed a routine of going to bed immediately after she got home at 4:00pm and slept until the following morning. In the end, she maxed out at 297 pounds. Even though she shed 50 pounds after joining law-enforcement services, she settled at around 250 pounds for nearly eight years.

The Breaking Point:

In 2011, Chloe separated from her husband, leaving her feeling like a complete failure. Her emotions were a reflection of her not taking care of herself and, as a result, she was miserable, working 70 hours a week to hide from the emptiness in her life.

While at home, she would drink whole bottles of wine with Chinese delivery 90 minutes before passing out most nights.

Six months later, she felt as if she would die if she couldn't change her lifestyle.

How She Lost It:

Chloe sought the services of a therapist and hired a personal trainer within a few months. She did all this because she believed she couldn't lose the weight on her own. She had issues with the tough love some trainers in her locality used during their training sessions. She couldn't work with these trainers because she needed someone that would partner with her and not yell at her.

Eventually, she found a perfect trainer. During the first session, he advised her that she needed to change her way of thinking if she wanted to experience long-term success with her weight loss. The trainer stopped her from speaking negatively about herself, including banning her from calling herself a fat chick any longer.

During the second week, the trainer taught her how to do simple five-minute meditation. She would take a few minutes break during the day just to be grateful for what she had, including her body that was supporting her to complete her work every day. Even though it felt like an effortless activity, setting aside five minutes every day to take care of herself was challenging. She had to confront how much she valued her work more than her well-being each time she meditated.

She then bought a notebook to record the BLTs she ate—bites, licks, and tastes. She did not look up calories or set any forbidden foods. Instead, she became aware of what she was eating. She would take the notebook to her trainer, who reviewed it regularly.

Because she respected him, she would avoid eating certain foods to avoid having to tell him! Whenever she over-ate, they would discuss together why and what she could have done instead. She realized that her trainer was more interested in her awareness of her triggers and dealing with why she was eating. He was not really bothered by whether she ate a cheeseburger or not.

By writing down every bite, she stopped herself from eating mindlessly. Instead, she had to pay attention to how much she ate so that she could record it accurately. This helped her get control of her appetite a lot sooner than she expected. The notebook also doubled up as her personal journal. She recorded her insecurities and the anger she felt toward her husband who had left her. Writing these feelings down gave her something else to do other than eat. This helped her to release those emotions so that she didn't need to bury them in food.

She started feeling better about herself and the choices made regarding her eating and fitness. She continued with physical exercise, and six months later, she had lost 80 pounds. By the end of the year, Chloe weighed 150 pounds, and her life was totally different!

KEY TAKEAWAYS

- There are at least nine different types of meditation. However, not all work for everyone, and you should find the one that works best for you.
- Meditation plays a critical role in the weight loss journey.
- Meditation works both on your physical and psychological being.
- You don't need sophisticated equipment to begin a regular meditation habit.
- Real life testimonies, backed by research studies, confirm that meditation for weight loss actually works.

Have you ever heard of positive affirmations for weight loss? Please move on to the next chapter for a more in-depth discussion of how affirmations will enhance your journey.

5

POSITIVE AFFIRMATIONS FOR WEIGHT LOSS

*S*tudies have revealed that when people are asked about things they want to change, weight loss is usually at the top of their to-do list. Some claim they want to do it to boost their self-esteem, and some want to improve their stamina, while others want to boost their immune system. There are many reasons to maintain a slimmer physique.

However, weight loss is not a walk in the park. And it is even more challenging to keep off the weight once you achieve your goal weight. If you have unsuccessfully tried several weight loss techniques, including those mentioned in the previous chapters, you're probably on the verge of giving up.

The good news is that you will have found the key to long-term weight loss if you can change your mindset. Although losing weight by thinking positively usually sounds too good to be true, success stories confirm that it is effective.

Using positive affirmations is a well-known technique that can help a person create a positive change in their life. The affirmations are positive statements that you say to yourself repetitively and with authority. Moreover, the statements can also help you increase your confidence when dealing with life situations and help you attain your goals.

Positive affirmations are used by many individuals that aim to attain fitness and weight goals. However, if you have tried to shed weight before, you will agree that sometimes it becomes exceedingly difficult to both stick to the plan and be positive. Sometimes the inability to stick to your schedule can lead to self-doubt. More often than not, you might start doubting your ability to succeed, which results in self-sabotage.

This is your chapter if you have been thinking about using positive affirmations in your weight loss journey. This chapter comprehensively breaks down the subject of positive affirmations and how they can help you throughout your journey. In addition, you will learn about the Law of attraction and why having a healthy mindset is essential. This chapter will also break down for you the meaning of self-love and why you are worth the time and the patience. As you keep reading, you will discover how you can change your emotional relationship with food. And we'll end with learning how to practice powerful positive affirmations. Let's kick off this exciting discussion by looking at the law of attraction.

LAW OF ATTRACTION

Simply put, the law of attraction is a viewpoint that states that positive thoughts bring positive results, while negative thoughts lead to adverse outcomes in your life. This law is based on the belief that thoughts are a form of energy. As a result, positive energy attracts success in all areas of your life, like relationships, health, and finances.

Advocates of the law of attraction argue that it is made up of central universal principles.

- **Like attracts like.** This principle states that people are likely to attract people who are similar to them. However, it also suggests that your thoughts also attract identical results. For instance, according to this principle, negative thinking will attract negative experiences while positive thinking will produce desirable experiences.
- **Nature hates a vacuum.** This principle of the

law of attraction states that when you get rid of negative things from your life, you make more room for more positive things to replace them. It is based on the philosophy that it is impossible to have an entirely empty space in your mind and life. Therefore, because there will always be something filling up this space, it is essential to fill it with positivity.

- **The present is always perfect.** This principle is based on the thought that there is always something you can do to improve the present moment. Even though the present might always seem flawed, this law suggests that instead of feeling anxious and miserable you should focus your energy on finding ways to make the present moment the best it possibly can be.

The law of attraction is always at work in our lives whether we are conscious about it or not. I usually think of the law of attraction as a strong helping hand. If you use this mighty helping hand the right way, you will be able to do the things you want in life, including weight loss. Another essential thing to note is that there are people that have instantly created some incredible things. However, in most cases, for most people, success is usually an ongoing, long-term process.

You should not think of the law of attraction as the magic fix-all that most people do. In my experience, I have seen many people get into problems by thinking that once they know about the law of attraction, their ideal life will magically manifest without putting any work in.

So why does it work instantly for some and take time for others? Well, most people have years of mental programming that go against the law of attraction. These individuals bear limiting beliefs about different things that keep them from manifesting the things they want simply because of a mental block.

Before we go any further, I need you to do me a favor. I would like you to think about the law of attraction as that mighty, helping hand we talked about. While the law of attraction is always at work in your life, there is a good chance you are not using it to its full potential.

How Do You Lose Weight Using the Law of Attraction?

Losing weight using the law of attraction works the same way as manifesting money. The only difference is that losing weight requires you to lose your excess pounds while getting rich requires gaining even more pounds to make you wealthy!

For you to lose weight, you must have a clear picture of what you want. For instance, I want to be skinny, is not a strong weight loss goal. You see, the universe doesn't know what being skinny looks like. So how will it determine how many pounds you want to lose?

Every person looks at the world through a different lens. Therefore, the universe cannot understand subjective terms like a little, a lot, fat, or skinny.

Here is how the Law of Attraction works:

Learn to define what you want to achieve precisely. The law of attraction will work perfectly for you if you are being as specific as possible. For example, you must define how many pounds you want to lose and the timeframe you wish to lose the weight in. After making that determination, take out your pen and write your exact goal. You can formulate your plan into several affirmations. For example:

- I am reaching my desired weight starting now.
- I currently weigh 120 pounds.
- I manifest my desired body.
- By December 2021, I will weigh 120 pounds.
- I am determined and willing to lose weight.
- My body is becoming stronger and healthy each day.

Alternatively, it can be in the form of a letter to yourself. For example, it could read like this:

I know my weight negatively affects my self-esteem, hinders me from doing a lot of things, and makes me less social. So I decided to work on myself, and I decided to learn my inner strength, beauty, and courage. By December 20, 2021, I will weigh 120 pounds. I will have higher self-esteem, and I will feel awesome in my own skin. I am thankful that I have the strength to make a change. I am grateful for my success in achieving my goal.

Reprogram your subconscious mind. Once you have determined the number of pounds you want to lose, and you see your future self in your mind's eye, you have already created the body you want to have. The body or ideal weight you desire now exists in your mind. This is the time to transform that body into its physical form.

Many people usually ask themselves about how they should get started. Immediately, thoughts of going into a caloric deficit, eating less, attending sports clubs, or running daily surface in their minds. The biggest mistake you can make is getting into things that promise weight loss. You start eating less and engaging in more sporting activities, but unfortunately, these programs are not long-lasting and neither will your progress be.

Your determinations will usually last a few weeks. You might lose a few pounds in the process but end up regaining them, or more, once you get tired of following the strict routines and meal plans.

Once you have decided to lose a definite number of pounds by a specific date, it is best to begin with small, decisive steps that include affirmations and visualization. Gradually, start getting yourself used to making positive affirmations at least twice a day, preferably in the morning and before you go to bed. You can repeat the positive affirmations whenever you have a moment to yourself.

Start with the visualization of your goals. Imagine yourself looking the way you aspire to, then start seeing yourself wearing that gorgeous small-sized dress. Picture yourself standing in front of your dressing mirror and telling yourself how proud you are of what you've achieved. Literally, feed your subconscious mind with positive affirmations and visualizations, as it will create a small space for positivity that will grow with time. Eventually, your subconscious will start helping you to lose weight naturally and effortlessly.

Your eating habits and relationships with food will change, and you will begin making better choices. For example, you will start to move around more so you can burn more calories. And whenever you eat something extra, you will not regret it because deep down, you know that you will not gain a single pound.

Avoid pushing yourself too much, but also don't limit yourself. Refrain from comparing yourself to other people and accept yourself as you are. If you can do this, then your weight loss journey will be effortless and exciting.

Useful Tips

You can do several things to learn how to apply the law of attraction in your life. Here are some ideas:

- **Start journaling.** Make it a habit to write your thoughts. This will help you to learn and recognize your habitual thought patterns better to see whether you are optimistic or pessimistic. And then you can learn more about changing the negative patterns you do see.
- **Create a mood board.** Make a visual reminder to help you maintain a positive mindset; stay motivated and focused on your goals.
- **Practice acceptance.** Quit focusing on what is wrong with the present or what you need to change. Instead, work on accepting things as they are. This does not mean that you will not keep

working hard toward a brighter future. It simply means that you won't be weighed down by wishing things were better right now.

- **Practice positive self-talk.** If you grapple with being excessively self-critical, set a goal to engage in positive self-talk daily. This will come much more easily with time, and you will find it harder to keep a negative mindset.

A HEALTHY MINDSET AND WHY YOUR MINDSET MATTERS

According to weight loss experts, in your weight loss journey, you should not only focus on your habits and behaviors but also focus on your mindset. While things like what you eat and how you move are essential, they argue that losing weight also requires mental health.

If you have been on the weight loss journey before, you might have discovered that the biggest challenge is gathering enough motivation to maintain a healthy weight. Therefore, it is imperative that you cultivate a weight loss mindset to increase your chances of succeeding.

So what is your current mindset? It is nothing but the perceptions and beliefs you have about yourself. Your view of yourself and the world influences your behavior, attitude, and outlook. For instance, if you believe you are likely to fail, there is a good chance that you will give up on your weight loss program when you hit roadblocks along the way. This is because self-defeating thought patterns can make weight loss management challenging.

On the other hand, if you believe that you can adapt to change and pick up new healthy ways of life successfully, you will succeed in your weight loss journey. Such a mindset is critical for diet motivation because it ensures that setbacks and struggles don't severely affect your journey and growth.

Behavioral experts suggest that your mindset plays a key role in changing your behavior. Luckily, your mindset is something that you can change and improve as soon as you are willing. They also reveal that if you can feel better about yourself and your environment, you will be more motivated to reach your goals and keep going when things get tough.

You must understand your mindset because it will go a long way in helping you improve your diet motivation.

How to Develop the Right Mindset for Weight Loss

Find positives in setbacks. Losing weight has many similarities to learning a new skill. Therefore, perfection is a fallacy! Getting used to a new habit will always be challenging, especially in the beginning. For instance, you might sleep through your alarm and miss an exercise session at times. Don't condemn yourself over it; just reschedule the missed session and make sure you do it better next time.

Also, whenever you are feeling stuck, ask for help. Studies reveal that structure and support play an essential role in someone's weight loss journey.

Don't think about weight, think about health. You can also develop the right mindset if you focus on your health rather than the number on the scale or the size of your jeans. This mindset shift will enable you to stick to your program and help you earn better results. Several studies have revealed that some subjects even performed meditation exercises, like yoga, to help them focus on their health instead of their weight. In the end, the ladies involved became more confident in losing weight and maintaining a healthy way of life.

Focus on the future. Sometimes you will experience tough days, and you might feel like giving up. When that happens, try to reflect on the reason you decided to make the change. For example, what motivated you to start this journey? You will need to know your weight loss why every time you need some extra motivation. Reminding yourself why you started the journey in the first place will give you the enthusiasm to keep going.

Patience. Human nature wants a quick fix for everything, especially in this era when everything happens almost instantaneously. However, things are a little different when it comes to weight loss. You will probably lose weight quickly during the first few months of your program. However, you're going to want to focus on the long-term to experience the best results.

In this regard, mindset will help to find a program that is realistic and sustainable for you. Moreover, it should fit your lifestyle. You don't have to get rid of a whole food group from your diet or deprive yourself.

Do it for personal reasons. It is more inspiring and rewarding to lose weight for yourself. The self-determination theory states that there are two types of motivators: intrinsic and extrinsic. Extrinsic goals are the ones motivated by external influences like social recognition and physical appearance. On the other hand, intrinsic goals tend to be more self-driven; examples of self-driven goals are better health and personal growth. According to studies, intrinsically motivated individuals find it more effortless to maintain their weight loss.

WHAT IT MEANS TO LOVE YOURSELF

Self-love is one of the most misunderstood concepts on the planet today. When you talk about self-love, many people shudder at the thought because they think about the self-centered and vain people they know about.

However, self-love is nothing like that; it is actually the opposite. True self-love is meek, restrained, and never blatant. You must be wondering how this helps in your weight loss journey because it creates some sort of dichotomy, right?

Well, you see, if you don't truly love yourself, then it will be challenging for you to do what is best for you, including caring for your body and shading weight. However, when you genuinely love yourself, you will want to take good care of yourself by eating right and exercising. You will respect yourself and expect others to respect you too.

How to Develop Self-Love

Step 1: Accept Yourself. Although you are in the process of improving your body through weight loss, it is also essential to accept yourself as you are at the beginning of the journey. It would be detrimental to complain about your body or put yourself down in any way.

Instead, your daily focus should be on accepting yourself completely, including your spirit, mind, and body. If it helps, you can even speak kindly to yourself using positive affirmations. You will learn about several positive affirmation statements later in this chapter.

Step 2: Be Gentle With Yourself. If you usually feel hostile and angry about yourself, and sometimes feel like your own enemy, you need to change that by making a conscious decision to treat yourself with dignity. For instance, stop being angry at your body because, quite frankly, it's the only thing keeping you alive.

You can't expect to change instantaneously. When you stop treating yourself like a naughty child, you will gradually discover how much better you feel about yourself.

Step 3: Feel the Love. It is not enough to go through the motions and say the words; you must also feel the love for yourself. As you vocalize your love for yourself, you need to focus on feeling that love. If you have never done this before, it may take a while to feel it, but once you get it right, the results are priceless.

Positive affirmations will help you develop self-love, which will go a long way to keeping you motivated during your journey.

CHANGING YOUR RELATIONSHIP WITH FOOD AND YOUR EMOTIONAL STATE

In your weight loss journey, the relationship you have with food matters a lot. A good relationship with food means having unconditional permission to eat the foods that make you feel great both mentally and physically. No foods should be off-limits, and you should not have intense emotional responses when you eat foods that are commonly labeled bad or good.

However, you cannot foster a good relationship with food overnight; it is something you have to work on your entire life. It can be similar to the way you work on your relationship with your partner or any other meaningful person in your life. Here is how you begin the journey of changing your relationship with food:

Understand Your Current Relationship With Food

Before you start working towards having a good relationship with food, it is important to identify the signs of a bad relationship with food. Remember, a good relationship with food has nothing to do with its quality or type. Instead, it is all about how you choose the foods you eat.

These are the signs of a bad relationship with food:

- You feel guilty about eating.
- You keep away from foods that you decided are bad for you.
- You have created a list of foods that you can and cannot eat.
- You depend on calorie counters and mobile apps to let you know when you are done eating for the day.
- You ignore your body's natural hunger signs.
- You have a history of using fad diets.
- You are usually stressed or anxious when eating in social gatherings because you fear what others will think of your food choices.

What Does a Good Relationship With Food Look Like?

Developing a good relationship with food is just like other relationships. It will take time, practice, and lots of patience. It is also critical to understand that your relationship with food goes beyond fueling your body. Humans are not like animals that eat for the sole reason of survival. Instead, we eat for several different reasons like pleasure, tradition, culture, and socialization.

If you begin to appreciate food as more than just a fuel source, you will start seeing the value in it and will be able to cultivate a healthier relationship.

These are signs that you have a good relationship with food:

- You have unconditional permission to eat the foods you enjoy.
- You pay attention to and respect your body's typical hunger cues.
- You eat when you are hungry and stop when you are full.
- There are no foods that are off-limits.
- You are not obsessed with the number on the scale.
- Other people's opinions don't dictate what you eat.
- You understand that the foods you eat don't define you.
- You moderately enjoy all foods.
- You go for the foods that make you feel best.
- Calories do not dictate your food choices.

If you are looking at the list above and wondering if you will ever get there, you are not alone. Many people find it hard to do away with the diet mentality. So don't focus on checking off every item on the list; just approach them one at a time and tackle them at your own pace.

How to Start Having a Good Relationship with Food

Instead of hoping for change, be proactive and make it happen. Remember that you are your own person. You have your history with food, personal preferences, and the right to go through this journey the way you want.

Use these helpful tips to get you started:

- **Give yourself unreserved authorization to eat.** Get rid of the restrictions you have around eating. Your body deserves to eat whenever you are feeling like you need to.
- **Eat when you are hungry.** Everyone has an inherent ability to regulate hunger. Forget about any diet culture that is controlling your eating and go back to learning and listening to natural hunger cues. This will make it easier for you to regulate your appetite and manage your food intake.
- **Practice mindful eating.** Mindful eating is when you eat in the moment and are totally conscious of the eating experience. It has emerged

as the cornerstone for fixing a lousy relationship with food.

- **Welcome all foods in your diet.** When you ascribe the label bad to a food, you give it unnecessary power. Therefore, try to start viewing all foods as equal, and over time, you will not feel the urge to overeat a particular food when it is around.

- **Mind your plate.** Don't justify your food choices. Instead, allow yourself to eat the food you feel is best for you at that particular moment.

- **Seek help from professionals.** Changing your relationship with food is a complex process, and you could use all the professional help you can get.

Practicing Powerful Positive Affirmations

While you should write your own positive affirmations to help in your weight loss journey, below is a list of positive affirmations related to weight loss and fitness that you can also use. It is important to note that positive affirmations are usually written and said in the present tense.

Here are positive affirmations you can practice saying:

- I am grateful for my body and how it knows what to do to keep me healthy.

- I love and accept myself.
- I make healthy choices daily that are good for my body and wellbeing.
- I embrace all positive behaviors and feelings surrounding food and food choices.
- My body is strong, and I enjoy exercising to stay healthy.
- I accept my body and am thankful for everything it has gotten me through.
- My body is an amazing machine, and I make choices that keep it healthy and strong.
- I am so happy to be me; I love and accept myself.
- I live a healthy lifestyle.
- I exercise because it makes me feel good.
- Every choice I make increases my wellbeing and health.
- I am an active person, and that helps me stay healthy.
- I love choosing nutritious foods that maximize my health and my body's functioning.
- I am healthier and stronger every day.
- It is easy for me to make healthy choices for my own body.
- I know how to provide my body with what it needs to be strong, healthy, and fit.
- I attract good things into my life.

- I am beautiful, smart, healthy, and good things come to me.
- I am lively and full of energy.
- My life is more appealing than my next meal.
- Unhealthy foods don't appeal to me. My body craves healthy, whole, and real food.
- Snacking and eating between meals is not profitable to me or my aspirations.
- I take a moment and assess the why before I give into cravings.
- Today I desire to heal and nourish my body.
- I am allied with my higher self.
- I'm an athlete capable of remarkable discipline.
- I value self-control and self-mastery over giving into pleasure and short-term impulses.
- I recognize what has not worked for me previously, and I have the guts to change.
- I have conquered my spontaneous nature and select food with purpose and integrity.
- I wake up every day with the apparent willpower to reach my ideal weight.
- Every time I stand firm against temptation, I reinforce my self-mastery.
- I don't judge myself against others. I'm on my own journey.

- I am strong enough to endure the bumps and bruises of life.
- I am fit, healthy, and full of energy.
- I let my journey be exclusive to me.
- Maintaining my ideal weight is effortless.
- I eat well, listen well, and live well.
- I admit that my thoughts are just thoughts. They are not real.
- I can be present. I only do one thing at a time.
- I turn daily tasks into mindful moments
- I defy my existing beliefs.
- I make peace with the past.
- I get outdoors and embrace the magnificence of nature.
- I savor every bite when I eat.
- My health, vitality, and energy increase with each breath I take.
- I think before I eat.
- All my cells are nourished by what I choose to eat.
- Every day brings me new hope.
- My will to live is more powerful than my craving.
- I find assurance in feeling healthy, vibrant, and strong.
- I enjoy moving my body and feeling my heart pumping.
- I think before I eat impulsively.

- My healthy habits are a part of the life that I live.
- I realize thoughts are just thoughts, and I can change them.
- I have an inner determination beyond food, weight, and the scale.
- Today, I choose to heal and nourish my body, mind, and spirit.
- I am creating a life of abundance.
- My purpose-filled life allows me to enjoy every moment.
- I am moving forward each day.
- I crave vegetables and whole foods to feel invigorated.
- I properly chew all the food that I eat, it gets digested properly, and this helps me reach my ideal weight.
- My metabolism is running at its best, helping me accomplish my desired weight.
- I let go of the guilt I have around food.
- I breathe in relaxation and breathe out stress.
- My journey is exceptional, and I do not compare myself to other people who are also losing weight.
- I drink plenty of water because it stirs up my metabolism and mood.
- My food choices are in line with my aspiration to be my best weight.

- I am eager to learn new things every day.
- I long for mindfulness each day.
- I am on a lifelong path of wellness. Every day I recommit to being my best self.

DOES THE POSITIVE AFFIRMATIONS TECHNIQUE WORK?

Case Study: Success Story

Here is the success story of someone who used positive affirmations to lose weight.

Rose was 235 pounds at the age of 14, which was tough on her. However, she never understood why she was so big. She believed that she was completely trapped in her body after unsuccessfully trying to lose weight. But luckily, she discovered that weight loss was not just about losing the pounds.

Rose was in her early twenties when she started learning about neuro-linguistic programming, NLP. The focus of NLP is the connection between our language, thoughts, and behavior. After she became qualified as an NLP coach, she had the opportunity to work on herself.

She started realizing that the primary culprit in the battle with her weight had always been her mindset and habits. She also realized that she needed to work on her self-esteem, self-acceptance, and happiness in her own skin. At first, she had thought that losing weight would give her those feelings. But she later realized that she needed to develop those feelings before she could start to lose the weight.

From her ongoing studies and practical NLP techniques, she discovered a lot about the subconscious mind and the significance of reframing negative self-talk. She also learned that everyone has patterns running in their subconscious minds that usually begin when they are young.

Rose discovered that we are heavily influenced by our family and friends and our surroundings. For example, if your parents used to give you chocolate to stop you from crying when you were young, there is a high likelihood that you have a deeply rooted attachment to chocolate. Moreover, you will associate it with making you feel better whenever you feel offended in your adult life. She also learned that the habits she learned when she was young protected her and made her unique. But some of the habits she picked were detrimental to her wellbeing and caused her to self-sabotage through emotional eating.

She sought professional help and discovered affirmations. Affirmations became an excellent way for her to send positive messages to her subconscious mind. After a few days, she started to think and behave with more acceptance toward herself.

She believes that she did not go from negative self-talk to self-love overnight—it took time. Her mindset had changed entirely, which set her off on a successful weight loss journey.

Here are the 15 affirmations she used:

- I believe in my ability to truly love myself for who I am. I accept my body's shape and acknowledge the beauty it holds.
- I am the creator of my future and the driver of my mind.
- I let go of unhelpful patterns of behavior around food.
- I allow myself to make choices and decisions for my higher good.
- I bring the qualities of fulfillment, happiness, and contentment into my life as I am now.
- I let go of any guilt I hold around my food choices.
- I accept my body for the shape I have been blessed with.
- I let go of relationships that are no longer for my benefit.
- I believe in myself and acknowledge my greatness.
- I allow myself to feel good being me.
- I accept myself for who I am.
- I bring the qualities of love into my heart.

- I have hope and certainty about the future.
- I am grateful for the body I own and all it does for me.

KEY TAKEAWAYS

- Your mindset plays a crucial role in your weight loss journey.
- The law of attraction can help you understand the importance of having the right attitude for your journey.
- Affirmations can help you develop the right mindset for your journey.
- Affirmations can guide you when changing your relationship with food.

In the next chapter, you will discover how you can develop fresh habits to help in your weight loss journey.

6

CHANGING HABITS FOR WEIGHT LOSS

CREATING HABITS FOR WEIGHT LOSS

By now, you have already learned a lot about how to lose weight. So far, we have established that losing weight is not about strict diets and gym routines. Based on the previous chapters, it is evident that even though diet and exercise are important, they might not be sustainable if done alone. According to remarks by various weight loss experts, to achieve healthy and sustainable weight loss, you also need to make several adjustments to your usual lifestyle. The key thing to remember is that weight loss is not a sprint; it is a marathon.

Many people fall for the fallacy that fad diets will have immediate results. However, studies have confirmed that most people who go that route usually fail. One nutritionist even revealed that some of the clients she had, who were using the popular diet plans, lost weight within a short period but gained it back quickly with some extra pounds to boot.

Please don't torture your body. There are better habits you can adopt to make your weight loss journey more interesting. As this chapter's title suggests, you can create lifestyle habits that will help you in your weight loss adventure. In this chapter, you will learn several tips you can use to make small but impactful changes to your weight loss adventure.

First, we will cover meaningful eating and how it differs from mindless eating. The chapter will also cover how you can practice mindful eating and how you create a routine. Other things we'll discuss here include portion control and how to set up your home kitchen.

As you keep reading, you will discover how you can set up your kitchen for success and the best way to deal with social situations. Dig in to find out how you can alter your routine for a successful weight loss endeavor.

MEANINGFUL EATING VS. MINDLESS EATING

What is Mindless Eating?

Mindless eating happens any time your brain is distracted and you are not conscious of what, or how much food you are consuming. Mindless eating is contributing significantly to the ever-expanding waistlines around the globe. Studies into mindful eating so far have focused on weight control and helping individuals develop healthier relationships with food. According to data from this research, five main factors can lead to mindless eating. They are:

- **Distracted Eating:** Mindless eating usually occurs when your mind is side tracked by distractions such as television, conversations, and phones.
- **Disinhibition:** This simply means eating even when you aren't hungry. For instance, you could start feeling bored and decide to eat food just to do something.
- **Lack of Awareness:** Do you know how easy it is for you to lose track of how much food you consume? This happens mostly when you are

eating out of a bag or not measuring out portion sizes.

- **External Reasons:** Sometimes an external source like a food advertisement or TV commercial could contribute to mindless eating. For instance, you could drive past a billboard with a juicy burger and immediately begin to crave it.

- **Emotional Eating:** Emotions also play a considerable role in mindless eating. Some people usually turn to food as a sense of comfort when they are sad—or may eat when they are feeling bored like we mentioned above. You should be attentive to your emotions and try not to feed them.

What Is Mindful Eating?

Mindful eating is keeping an in-the-moment awareness of food and drink as you consume it. It usually involves observing how the food makes you feel and the signals your body sends about taste, satisfaction, and fullness.

Mindful eating requires individuals to acknowledge and accept their feelings instead of judging those feelings, thoughts, and other bodily sensations. It can extend to include the process of buying, preparing, and serving your food before you eat it.

For many people, their busy daily lives usually make their mealtimes rushed affairs. Most of the time, you could find yourself eating in your car as you commute to work or at your desk in front of your computer monitor. As a result, you end up eating mindlessly, shoveling food down without regard to whether you are still hungry or not.

Mindful eating does not mean being perfect or eating the right things all the time. It is also not about establishing stringent rules for the number of calories you can eat or which foods you have to include, or avoid, in your diet. Instead, it is about focusing all your senses on being present while you shop for, prepare, serve, and eat food.

While mindful eating is not for everyone, many people find that by eating mindfully, even for only a few meals per week, helps them become more accustomed to your body. As a result, you will avoid overeating, which makes it easier for you to improve your dietetic habits.

What Are the Benefits of Mindful Eating?

Paying attention to how you feel while you eat will help you learn how to appreciate your food and the experience of eating. Some things to focus on are the food's texture, the taste of each bite, and your body's level of hunger and fullness signals. You should also focus on how different foods affect your mood and energy levels.

Here are some of the benefits you get from eating mindfully:

- It helps you to slow down and take a break from the daily hustle and bustle, which reduces stress and anxiety.
- It also helps you observe and change your relationship with food. This will help you find out when you are eating for reasons other than hunger.
- It also enables you to experience a greater pleasure from the food you consume as you learn how to slow down and better appreciate each meal.
- You can also make healthier choices about what you eat by finding a pattern in how different types of food make you feel after you eat them.
- Studies have revealed that you can improve your digestion by being mindful of what you eat.
- Eating mindfully also helps you to feel fuller more quickly and consume less.
- You will also develop a better connection with where your food came from, and the journey it takes to your plate.
- Finally, it also makes you eat in a consistent and more balanced manner.

How to Practice Mindful Eating

Mindfulness in general requires you to participate in an activity with complete awareness. For mindful eating, it is critical that you eat with all your attention rather than on autopilot as you watch your favorite TV show or chat with your friends. If your attention does go astray, please bring it back gently to your food and work to savor the entire experience.

When you are getting started, try practicing mindful eating for short, five-minute sessions and slowly build up from there. It is also important to note that you should begin the act of mindful eating when making your shopping list or checking the menu in a restaurant.

Here are some tips on how you can practice mindful eating:

- Start by taking several deep breaths and consider the nutritional value of each piece of food. There are many different suggestions from different dietitians regarding which foods are healthy and which ones are not. The best rule of thumb is to ensure you eat food that is as close to its natural form as possible.
- Make use of all your senses when you are shopping, cooking, serving, and eating food. Pay attention to how different foods look, smell, and feel as you

prepare them. Additionally, you should make a point to hear how the food sounds as you cook it and how it tastes when you eat it.

- Use your observation skills and curiosity to be aware of yourself and of the food you are eating. Ensure you are sitting in a relaxed posture, and acknowledge your surroundings so you can eliminate any distractions. If you focus on what is happening around you it will take away from the mindful eating experience.

- Be in tune with your hunger. How hungry are you? You should come to the table when you are hungry and not feeling starved after you've missed several meals. It is also important to know your intentions for every meal. Are you eating because of hunger, or is it because you are bored or need a distraction?

- Always take a moment to appreciate the food that is in front of you. You should also be conscious of the people you are sharing the meal with before you begin eating. The things you should focus on include the texture, shape, smell, and color of the food. Pay attention to your reaction to the food and how the smell makes you feel.

- As you take a bite, take a moment to note how it feels in your mouth. How would you describe each food's texture? Can you identify all the ingredients and the different flavors? Ensure you chew systematically and take note of how you chew.

- Put your spoon or fork down between bites. Before you pick it back up to continue, take a few moments to consider how you feel. Are you still hungry, or do you feel satiated? Listen to your stomach and your body, not the food on your plate. Learn to know when you are full and when you should stop eating.

- Be thankful for and reflect on where the food came from. Reflect on the animals and plants involved and all the people who took part in transporting it to reach your plate. When you are mindful of the origins of your food, it becomes easier to make wiser and more sustainable selections.

- Keep eating slowly as you converse with your dining companions. Please pay attention to your body's signals of fullness. If you are dining solo, do your best to be present for the experience of eating the food.

How to Fit Mindful Eating Into Your Life

Most of the people I have talked to usually think it isn't practical for them to be mindful of every bite they take. They claim that the pressures of life usually force them to eat on the go. Or that they only have a limited window of time to have a meal or risk going hungry for the rest of the day. Are you in the same predicament?

Well, even if you cannot follow mindful eating strictly, you can still avoid eating mindlessly. You can also avoid ignoring the signals your body is sending. For example, you can take a few deep breaths before you eat your next meal or snack. This will help you to reflect on what you are about to consume quietly. It will help you decide whether you are eating to resolve hunger or respond to an emotional trigger.

You will be able to determine whether the food you are eating is nutritionally healthy or emotionally comforting. Even if you are forced to eat at your desk, please take a moment to focus fully on the food. It is advisable to avoid multitasking or doing anything on your computer or phone while you eat.

This will help if you think of mindful eating as exercising— every little bit counts. The bottom line is slowing down as much as you can, focusing on the process of eating and being attentive to your body signals. When you do this, you will experience greater satisfaction from your food, and you will have better control over your diet and nutritional habits.

Switching from Mindless Eating to Mindful Eating

I know you are thinking to yourself that all this sounds great, but how do you make the switch? I have you covered! Here are some areas to address to help you make the switch:

Mindless Eating	Mindful Eating
Instead of multitasking while eating, like watching TV or driving while you eat.	Focus all your attention on the food before you, and relish the experience.
Instead of eating to satisfy an emotional need, like eating because you are lonely or bored.	Eat only to satisfy physical hunger.
Instead of eating junk or comfort food.	Eat meals and snacks that are nutritionally healthy.
Instead of eating meals as quickly as you can.	Take it slow and savor every bite of your food.
Instead of eating to finish all the food on your plate.	Stop eating once you feel full.
Instead of ignoring your body signals of fullness.	Pay attention to the feeling of your stomach and your hunger levels.

HOW TO USE MINDFULNESS TO INVESTIGATE YOUR RELATIONSHIP WITH FOOD

Whether you are conscious about it or not, food significantly affects your wellbeing. Food can affect how you feel physically and even evoke an emotional response. Additionally, it can affect your energy levels or drain your energy resources, making you feel moody and gloomy.

It is common knowledge that eating more fruits and vegetables, and less processed foods and sugar, is better for your health. However, if we only needed the knowledge of what is healthy, then the world wouldn't be laden with overweight issues and addiction to junk foods.

Eating mindfully helps you to be attuned to your body, making it easy for you to recognize how different foods affect you emotionally, physically, and mentally. Such knowledge is key in helping you make the switch to better foods. For instance, if you discover that the sugary snack you usually crave when you feel tired makes you feel worse, it becomes effortless to manage that craving and opt for an option that boosts your energy and mood.

Many people only pay attention to how food makes them feel if it causes them any physical discomfort. Experts suggest that instead of asking whether your food makes you sick, you should ask how good your food will make you feel. Consider how energized and enthusiastic you will feel after having a particular snack or meal.

How Does Your Food Make You Feel?

To properly investigate your relationship with food, it is critical to know how different foods make you feel. Take note of how you feel when you swallow the food, and how you feel a few hours after taking the food.

Here is a simple exercise to help you track the relationship between what you eat and how it makes you feel:

1. Eat in your normal fashion. Choose the foods, amounts, and times you usually eat. The only thing you will add is a conscious attitude of what you are doing.
2. Record everything you eat, including nibbles and snacks you take in between meals. Don't delude yourself; you are not going to remember everything unless you write it down.
3. Be mindful of your physical and emotional feelings. Take note of how you feel five minutes, one hour, or two hours after taking a particular meal.
4. Be attentive and find out if a shift or physical change follows the eating of any food. How are you feeling? Are you feeling better or worse than you felt before eating? Are you feeling tired or energized? Are you sluggish or alert?

Keeping these records will help increase your consciousness of how particular meals and snacks affect you emotionally and physically.

Experiment With Diverse Food Combinations

If you can connect your food choices to your physical and mental wellbeing, the food selection process becomes a matter of listening to your body. For example, you might discover that eating carbohydrates makes you feel heavy and weary for long hours. As a result, you will be more inclined toward low-carb meals.

However, different foods affect people in different ways. So, it may take some trial and error to discover which foods and combinations are ideal for you. Here is a simple exercise to help you realize how various food combinations and quantities impact your wellbeing.

- Start experimenting with your food:
- You can try eating less food more often.
- If you eat a lot of meat, try going for three days without eating any kind of meat.
- Alternatively, you can exclude red meat and include white meat like fish and chicken.
- Exclude certain foods from your meals one at a time and observe how you feel afterward. For example, try cutting out (or limiting) sugar, salt, bread, or coffee intake.
- Play around with various food combinations. Try

eating starch meals only, or proteins and fruits at the same time, or all vegetable meals.

- Record everything you observe as you experiment with your eating routine. You will be seeking out the eating patterns that add to the quality of your life and which ones take away some quality.

- Keep on experimenting with various food types, combinations, and quantities for a few weeks. Ensure you keep track of your physical, mental, and emotional feelings.

SETTING UP YOUR HOME AND KITCHEN FOR SUCCESS

What are your childhood kitchen memories like? Did you help your mom cook? Or are you the type that just stood there with eyes and nostrils waiting to see and smell everything being cooked? These memories are what will shape your perception of the kitchen into adulthood. My childhood memories make me see the kitchen as a place where the family gathers to experience laughter, cooking, and eating together. How do your memories shape your view of the kitchen?

For me, it can be the perfect room for meditation. However, to develop mindfulness as you cook, you need to have everything in the right order. The first step is setting up a mindful kitchen. In an ideal situation, you ought to have everything you need to prepare a particular meal. For instance, you should have all your ingredients measured, all of your equipment ready, and if you are a music fan, your favorite music playing in the background. As you go through the cooking process, stay connected with the ingredients, honor their presence, and enjoy your time in the kitchen.

If you want success with mindful eating, you have to make it happen. Here are some tips to help you set up your home and kitchen for success:

Swap Your Dishes

Consider replacing your 12-inch plates with smaller dinner plates. Studies have revealed that you are more likely to over-serve yourself if you are using a large plate. The same studies also suggest that even a two-inch difference in the size of dinner plates resulted in 22% fewer calories served. Suppose a normal dinner plate bears 800 calories; using a smaller plate alone could help you lose approximately 18 pounds per year.

Change the Color of Your Dishes

If you change the color of your dishes, it could affect your level of intake by changing how the amount of food appears. According to research, when you use a dish that offers more contrast with the food, it reduces the amount you serve by 21%. This is because a higher contrast between the plate and the food makes your serving look bigger.

Develop Workplace Wellness

Many studies have concluded that people lose weight during weekdays but gain weight over the weekends. These studies also hint that people who lose weight during weekdays usually maintain a healthy weight in the long run. Therefore, it would even help if you set up a healthy environment at your workplace that will help you eat healthier meals just between Monday and Friday.

Invest in Measuring Cups and Spoons

Measuring tools help you understand what a portion looks like, helping you to avoid overeating. If you don't have them, pause right here and go get some! One set is enough.

Hide the Sugary Stuff from View

If you love chocolate and you can't stop yourself when they are in plain sight, it is time to do something about it. A study on this matter revealed that the people who had candy on their desks ended up eating three times more than the volunteers who hid candy containers in their desks. In addition, they ate six times more candy than those who had to walk a short distance to buy the candy.

Using the same principle, keep unhealthy snacks out of your house. Whenever you feel like having a cookie, go to the bakery and buy just one to avoid the temptation of eating a whole package.

Organize Your Fridge for Success

When you rush home from work feeling very hungry, chances are you will grab the first snack you come across in your house. So make sure the first snack you grab is a good one by putting healthy choices in clear containers at the front of the fridge. On the other hand, hide all the less healthy options in opaque containers at the back. For example, you can place baggies and containers with fresh fruits, and yogurt near the front of the fridge to make the choice fast and easy.

Prepare Portion-Controlled Ready-to-Eat Snacks

Having a treat once in a while doesn't have to sabotage your diet. You can do some quick preparations to avoid sitting down with the family-size portion of something when you want to grab a snack. Once you get home from your grocery-shopping, portion your snacks into smaller containers so that you can quickly grab one and indulge without feeling guilty.

Make Your Kitchen a No-Phone Zone

According to studies, the average American spends around 10 hours a day glued to some type of screen. However, you can make eating your reason to escape. If you eat while distracted on your phone, you are likely to ignore your body's hunger and satiety signals and end up overeating.

HOW TO APPROACH SOCIAL SITUATIONS

Social events and eating go hand in hand. These events can also cause a lot of stress and anxiety around eating. As a matter of fact, some people avoid social events entirely because they fear the events could veer them off a certain diet. They believe they could end up consuming too much of the wrong food.

However, with several reminders and guidelines, you can learn how to enjoy the good things that a social event offers without arousing the pre-event anxiety and post-event stomach upset. Here are some tips that will come in handy:

Practice in Several Social Events

Practice doing a mindful check-in. Gently focus on your intentions and goals to help you make choices. During special occasions, celebrations, and holidays you are allowed to have fun, celebrate, and not have to worry about your choices.

Here's how you can enjoy special events and still make healthy choices:

- Don't go to social events on an empty stomach to avoid being blindsided by your stomach. Before leaving for the event, eat a healthy snack. This will keep you just full enough to keep you from making an unhealthy choice once you arrive.
- Beware of the foods that really call to you. Try new dishes and tastes instead.
- Learn to tune into your hunger and satiety levels to make appropriate choices.
- Once you have had enough to feel full, stay away from the food tables.
- You can hold a partially filled plate or a cup as you interact with others if that helps.
- Finally, remember that you don't have to clear everything from your plate.

Remain Mindful as You Interact with Others

You can enjoy your meals, remain attuned, and be social all at the same time. Social eating is a daily reality for most people. If it is for you too, here are some tips:

- When eating with your colleagues or family members, practice being present in the conversations.
- Frequently switch your attention to your body and your experience eating. Take note of how hungry or full you feel and the food tastes. Allow your sensory experience to keep you grounded in the act of eating. Stay focused on that for a little while.
- Then switch back to the social setting. Focus on the discussion, listening, and contributing mindfully. Repeat this throughout the social sitting.

Mindful Eating in Restaurants

It is easy to eat too much or order foods that don't support your health at restaurants. Do you eat out frequently or just every once in a while? Regardless of your restaurant routine, here are useful tips to consider:

- Go through the menu beforehand and check out the options you have.

- It would help to forego the "extras" like desserts and appetizers and stick to the main course.
- Ask for sauces and dressings on the side to help control how much is served.
- You don't have to finish all the food on your plate. You can pack up the rest to take home once you feel physically full.
- Remember the tips for mindful social engagement and mindful eating.

LIST OF SUSTAINABLE MINI HABITS THAT WILL CHANGE YOUR LIFE

Several studies and personal experiences have confirmed that small steps can get you far in life. The secret is making the small steps consistently in the right direction. While building a big habit can be a tall order, building a small habit is much more straightforward.

In this section, you will learn a few habits that will practically change your life.

- Drink a glass of water first thing every morning. The nature of our busy schedules usually denies us the opportunity to get enough water throughout the day. More often than not, we also find ourselves replenishing with tea, coffee, or soda.

Learn to drink a glass full of water every morning when you wake up.

- Park as far away from the door as possible. Try to make your lifestyle less sedentary by finding easy ways to take more steps each day. In this regard, simple steps from your car to the office are an improvement.
- All your meals should include raw fruit and/or vegetables.
- After every hour, get up from your desk and stretch. Sitting for long hours is not good for your body or your brain.
- Carry protein-rich snacks everywhere you go. These snacks will help you avoid the hunger levels that would normally push you into eating the first thing you find. Remember, protein is satiating and will keep you fuller for longer.

DOES MINDFUL EATING WORK?

Many success stories confirm that mindful eating can change your life for the better. Here is one that particularly caught my attention:

Name: Tasha

Tasha revealed that she had struggled with her weight for most of her life. She was never in an active weight loss mode, and never achieved her goal weight—even after trying many different approaches. According to her, she was moving from one extreme to the other.

Childhood: Tasha had been self-conscious about her weight for as long as she could remember. During a pool party in the seventh grade, she realized she was heavier than her friends.

The boys in the neighborhood made fun of her thick legs. However, this did not stop her from going out with her friends and participating in other activities. But she was always conscious of her weight and wished she was thinner. When she transitioned to college, she gained more interest in dieting and nutrition. The irony is that she also gained more weight during this period, even while researching weight loss and getting to understand different philosophies around weight loss.

She moved to the dorms with unlimited cafeteria food, studied a lot, and had poor sleeping habits. She worked as a hostess and enjoyed eating cheesy sandwiches and peanut butter pie—and ended up weighing around 160 pounds.

When her brother got engaged, she got fitted for her brides-maid's dress, and you guessed right! By the time the wedding was approaching, the dress no longer fit.

A wake-up call: This was a wake-up call for her, and she started pursuing dieting ideas. Her first diet book focused on a low-fat diet. With this new routine, she lost a modest amount of weight that made her feel just okay about her body. However, it wasn't like she felt comfortable wearing a bathing suit in front of people. She claims that she was 10 pounds shy of her dream weight. However, she slaved away in deprivation and frustration for 20 years to get there.

Diet after diet: She used to spend money on any promising diet she would come across. After working really hard to commit to the diets, she would only lose 2 to 3 pounds. The lack of progress would frustrate her, and she would go hunting for a new plan.

She hired coaches, counted calories, downloaded hypnosis tracks, and tried all kinds of diets. It was so much that weight loss had become a full-time job for her.

The turning point: The final diet she tried was zero sugar. It was her turning point in her weight loss journey. After going 30 days without sugar, Tasha gained 5 more pounds. And, if that was not enough, she broke out in acne even after the book she was following promised she would have clear skin.

The experts claimed all her cravings to overeat would go away if she eliminated sugar from her diet. In Tasha's case, the opposite was true as she overate all of the other foods she loved. At this point, she decided to find out why she couldn't stop eating.

The mental pivot: Tasha's mindset toward weight loss changed. Previously, her mindset was that her weight was unfair. But she decided to embrace this journey instead of resenting it. She claims that at this point, she had to decide that the weight loss journey was the good part. That the blessing of developing a fit body was in the process, and discovered that the joy was in doing the work, not reaching the destination.

She found out why she ate too much: At this point, she started paying attention to her behavior around food. As she began doing this, things started to change. For instance, she realized that she didn't like some of the foods she thought she did. She also realized that she wasn't paying attention to how much she ate, and the more distracted she was while eating, the more she ate. She had mindless eating habits like scrolling through social media during breakfast.

Then stumbled into mindful eating: She realized that eating with mindfulness and intentionality while tracking what she ate had become her new goal. She claims that shifting her weight loss efforts to *process-based* goals instead of *results-based* goals made all the difference. It was clear to her now, and she decided to enjoy the process rather than sweat for the results.

Here are the strategies she embraced to lose those last 10 pounds:

- She established three periods during her day to intentionally and purposefully eat.
- She limited mealtime distractions.
- She started chewing slowly and savoring every bite.
- She also put her fork down between bites.
- Finally, she started checking in with her body mid-meal and realized she often didn't have to finish all of the food on her plate.

KEY TAKEAWAYS

- It is possible to create new habits to aid your weight loss journey.
- Breaking mindless eating habits and developing mindful eating habits is not difficult.

- How you set up your home, especially your kitchen, will help you to succeed.
- You don't have to stay away from social events when working on your healthy weight.
- It is all about the little things you do, not the big ones!

Now that you know how to create new habits for your weight loss journey, it's time to take it to the next level. Please move to the next chapter to discover how you can get —and maintain—motivation for weight loss.

7

MOTIVATION FOR WEIGHT LOSS

*S*tarting your weight loss journey is usually the easier part. However, sticking to your plan sometimes feels impossible. On many occasions, people lack the motivation to get started, or when they do get started, they seem to lose the motivation soon after.

If you have been struggling to stay motivated during your weight loss journey, today is your lucky day! First, you will be happy to hear that motivation is something you can work on. This chapter covers in-depth how you can garner motivation through every stage of your journey.

The first part of the chapter will break down the different types of motivation. After that, you will learn several tips that you can use to foster motivation in your weight loss journey. Getting motivated can sometimes be easier than maintaining it. Because of this, I have an entire section dedicated to enlightening you on how to maintain sustainable motivation.

TYPES OF MOTIVATION

The best way to find the motivation you require is to figure out where to look. You have to look both outside yourself and inside yourself. Sounds simple, right?

You will need two kinds of motivation: intrinsic and extrinsic. Extrinsic motivation is the inspiration you get from external sources. For example, your trusted physician can encourage you, or you could be motivated to lose weight out of fear of having poor health. Also, motivation to lose weight in order to fit in that flattering outfit is extrinsic as well.

On the other hand, intrinsic motivation emanates from within. If your motivation to lose weight is the sense of accomplishment you get after finishing your workout session, then your source of motivation is intrinsic. If you go for a healthy snack because it makes you feel better about your choices, your motivation comes from within.

In a nutshell, you can think of extrinsic motivation as when you are motivated to lose weight because of a reward (wearing those pants) or to avoid punishment (poor health), while intrinsic motivation is when you are motivated to lose weight because of personal rewards like the feeling you experience.

I know you are wondering why you need both types of motivation in your weight loss journey. As you keep reading, you will realize that intrinsic and extrinsic inspiration come into play at different times in your adventure. Therefore, if you understand how the two forms of motivation work together, you will be well equipped with the tools you require to battle roadblocks.

HOW NORMAL MOTIVATION DEVELOPS

When children are born, they have intrinsic motivation. In their childhood, they explore their surroundings and discover their ability to enjoy and gain personal satisfaction. With time, these explorations are quickly paired with external motivators like encouragement from parents and guardians. This is a fundamental part of a child's development because they need to learn a lot of things and must take risks to do that.

If they are not encouraged, they might lack the motivation to take part in the necessary journey of discovery. If you take a look at children between one and three years old, you will realize that they have a particular pattern of exploration where they use their parents as the home base in their adventures.

The children will often go check things out but consistently go back to their parents for additional encouragement. In this process, the children develop both intrinsic and extrinsic motivation. In the course of typical child development, the children find the balance between the two types. If there is no proper balance, the children will find it difficult to complete more challenging tasks.

For example, if a child does not respond to external motivators well and they have to do something undesirable, that child is not likely to complete the desired behavior. This is also true for employees. An individual may find it difficult to keep a job if they do not desire the boss's approval, don't need the money, or do not receive any personal satisfaction from the job. This kind of person lacks both intrinsic and extrinsic motivation.

What makes it difficult to develop the right balance between intrinsic and extrinsic motivation?

Fearful and Overprotective Parents

If a parent overprotects their child, they will learn that the world is a dangerous place and they shouldn't take risks. However, as discussed earlier, the world's natural pattern of development through exploration requires the ability to take risks. Suppose the child becomes too fearful; they learn to disregard internal motivators of inquisitiveness and self-motivation. As a result, the child avoids unfamiliar tasks or situations that could lead to possible failure or discomfort. Consequently, the only tasks the child will be willing to pursue are those approved by the parent.

Later, when such a child grows up, they will continue being dependent on external motivators like their spouse, boss, or coach to encourage them to go after their dreams because of their fear of failure.

Non-Specific Response

Parents misguidedly offer their children non-specific, positive encouragement, believing it will help build internal motivation. For example, if you tell your child, you are so smart, or you are great at sports, you're not being specific enough to instigate positive, extrinsic benefits in their lives.

Instead of using non-specific sentiments like those shared above, you could say:

Your research paper is excellent because you thoroughly researched before you started writing.

Or, I can see you are practicing your ball control because you can dribble better.

When you give your child any kind of feedback, ensure it is tied to the efforts and behaviors they have control over. On the contrary, non-specific feedback normally targets factors that may not be in the person's control. As a result, less goal-oriented behaviors may become the preferred outcome. Can being "smart" inspire a person? Actually, it is more likely to have the opposite effect. The individual will ask themselves, is there a need for me to keep studying when I am already smart?

Focus on Rewards

Many times, people use external rewards as inspiration, which normally provokes the need for constant extrinsic motivation. For instance, if a school offers children 100 USD as a reward for perfect school attendance, the children will likely be motivated to attend school just to get paid. And then if the school changed its policy later and stopped paying for attendance, children will lose their motivation to attend.

Based on the example above, we can conclude that if children keep getting rewards for activities, they will likely find it difficult to set or achieve any goals without external motivation. The child should be motivated to go to summer school because the classes themselves are enjoyable.

WHY TOO MUCH RELIANCE ON EXTRINSIC MOTIVATION IS PROBLEMATIC

Incapability to Set and Attain Independent Goals

If you have followed this discussion so far, you know that a person who relies heavily on external motivation will only achieve goals and follow instructions set by others. If people don't have high enough levels of intrinsic motivation, they might not be able to set and attain personal goals without external forces pushing them. Although someone may do well as an employee under a structured work environment, they may not follow through with their self-improvement goals like weight loss.

External vs. Internal Validation

External and internal validation are closely related concepts. External validation is when you need another person or something else to confirm your value. This could be valuing yourself by the salary you get or placing your value on what someone else says about you. The need for validation is a problem because of the effect it has on your self-esteem. You see, if you cannot always get outside approval, you will become unhappy with yourself whenever it is not readily available.

On the flip side, internal validation is your ability to feel good about your efforts and progress—even those other people may not see as worthwhile. For example, someone attending therapy sessions could be making cognitive changes that will lead to lasting behavioral changes. But, since these changes are not visible to the outside world, people close to them might not be able to see the useful skills that are being developed. If that person values what the others can observe, they may quit the therapy sessions even though the changes were happening.

HOW DOES SOMEONE DEVELOP INTRINSIC MOTIVATION?

Develop Internal Rewards

If you find yourself overly reliant on external motivation, you can develop intrinsic motivation by tying internal rewards to external motivators. For instance, if you desire to lose weight and find that being part of a weight loss support group is helpful, use that external motivator to develop and discover internal rewards.

As you start losing weight because of the external motivators, shift your focus to how excellent you feel physically as you lose weight. Let your focus be on the idea that you are losing weight thanks to the efforts that you are putting in.

Try to identify specific changes that you have made and pat yourself on the back for carrying through with those habits.

Precise Positive Feedback

It will also help if you are specific with the positive feedback you give yourself. Studies have confirmed that most people who rely on extrinsic motivation are usually very negligent in providing themselves with feedback. The ideal move would be to keep a notebook and record all self-statements regarding the goals that you are striving for. After that, review the statements on your list and mark each of them as either positive or negative.

If you are an externally motivated person, you will likely have more negative self-statements. You will realize that your negative self-statements are mostly specific while your positive self-statements are far less specific. For that reason, you will need to put more effort into ensuring that you are being more specific with your positive self-statements to develop more intrinsic motivations.

EXTRINSIC MOTIVATION TO LOSE WEIGHT

In many cases, individuals start a weight loss program because of extrinsic reasons. For example, their clothes no longer fit them, their doctor has advised them to do so, or because of pressure from loved ones. Make no mistake; these external factors go a long way in helping you to get started.

Whenever you feel external pressure to lose weight, allow it to motivate you to collect information. It might be too early for you to start a program, but you can gather information about weight loss plans and exercise routines. Try to find out if there are small steps you can take to improve your health before you embark on a program. You can also consult your physician to learn more about making small changes to your diet that could affect your health.

Extrinsic motivation can also come in handy when you need a gentle push to accomplish short-term goals. For example, you might be fully aware of the benefits of exercising, including how good it makes you feel, but still struggle to go to the gym. In such cases, promise yourself healthy rewards for reaching specific habit milestones.

However, extrinsic motivation can become a bad thing if you use it as your primary motivation for long-term goals. Please don't fall into the trap of losing weight solely for aesthetic reasons. Your only concern shouldn't be to look good. I am not saying that looking sexy is not good, but l am saying that you shouldn't commit to weight loss purely because of external motivation . . . it will end in tears.

INTRINSIC MOTIVATION TO LOSE WEIGHT

When you talk to weight loss experts, you will learn that people who are successful in their journey are normally motivated by intrinsic factors. For example, they feel good when they exercise and practice other healthy habits.

Here are three, simple steps to help you enhance your internal motivation to lose weight:

- **Set short-term goals** – You will be setting yourself up for success if you come up with short–term, practicable goals. For example, your long-term goal might be to lose 20 pounds. But your complimentary, short-term goal might be something like eating a lean, healthy breakfast every day.
- **Keep a journal** – Jot down all of your goals in a journal. At the end of each day, comment on the day's success. Remember, just taking the time and writing it down in your journal is an achievement in itself. Always use positive words to express how you feel about your weight loss actions.
- **Acknowledge your success** – Take some time to evaluate your success and give yourself credit for your accomplishment. Review your journal

regularly and be proud of every step you take
toward improving your health.

The discussion above shows that both kinds of motivation play a key role in the weight loss journey. Extrinsic motivation is important when you are dealing with short-term goals and need quick bursts of motivation. However, external motivation cannot help you stay on course. Intrinsic motivation is what will help you follow through with your long-term, weight loss aspirations. Therefore, if you can use the two appropriately, you will have a constant cycle of motivation to push you toward your overall goals.

HOW TO CREATE SUSTAINABLE MOTIVATION FOR WEIGHT LOSS

Now that you are aware of the two types of motivation, you are in a better place to create your own motivation. Here are some ways you can motivate yourself to lose weight:

Establish Why You Want to Lose Weight

Plainly describe all of the reasons you want to lose weight and write them down. This will help you to remain committed and motivated to attain your goals. Make an effort to go through them each day to act as a reminder whenever you are tempted to deviate from your weight loss plans.

Your motivation could be to prevent diabetes, to look good for your wedding, or to improve self-esteem. Studies show that people motivated by internal reasons tend to be more successful than those motivated by external factors alone.

Focus on Process Goals

Most people in weight loss programs only set outcome goals for the weight they want to be at the end of it all. But when you focus on outcome-based goals, you may end up derailing your motivation. They often feel too distant and might even leave you feeling beleaguered.

As an alternative, consider setting process-based goals. This includes the actions you are going to commit to so that you can attain your goals. For instance, your process-based goal could be to exercise four times a week. According to studies, overweight women specifically who focus on process-based goals are more likely to lose weight and less likely to diverge from their diets.

It is advisable to have SMART goals—they should be Specific, Measurable, Achievable, Realistic, and Time-based. Examples of SMART goals include:

- I will walk quickly for 25 minutes today.

- I will eat four servings of vegetables every day this week.
- I will only drink one soda this week.

Have Practical Expectations

If you browse through the internet, you will find multiple diets and diet products that claim quick and effortless weight loss. Nevertheless, many experts recommend that you should only lose around 1 to 2 pounds weekly.

When you set unachievable goals, you are setting yourself up for failure. You will end up frustrated when you don't achieve those goals and give up. Alternatively, if you set and attain achievable goals, you will end up having a feeling of accomplishment. Studies also confirm that individuals who reach their self-determined goals are more likely to stay on course throughout the duration of their journey.

Go For a Plan that Aligns with Your Lifestyle

It would be best to select a weight loss plan that you can stick to. It is not advisable to go for a plan that is almost impossible to follow successfully in the long term. Most diets are based on reducing calorie intake. Reducing your calorie intake will result in weight loss. However, dieting—particularly yo-yo dieting—is said to be a predictor of future weight gain. Because of this, you should avoid strict diets that eliminate certain foods. Studies have revealed that you are less likely to lose weight if you use an all-or-nothing approach. As an alternative, consider developing your own tailored plan. Your plan should at least have these habits that are proven to be effective:

- Decrease your calorie intake.
- Reduce portion sizes.
- Reduce the frequency of snacks.
- Reduce fried foods.
- Eat plenty of vegetables.

Find Social Support

We all need regular support and positive feedback to stay motivated. Share your weight loss goals with family and friends so they can provide you with support throughout the journey. Many people also find it beneficial to have a weight loss buddy with whom they work out. You can also hold each other accountable and encourage each other throughout the journey.

Apart from a partner, it would help if you also got support from your usual friends. It is also advisable to join a support group; it could be an in-person or an online support group. I have found all of these types of support to be profitable.

Have a Weight loss Journal

Monitoring and regularly evaluating yourself is a critical part of weight loss motivation and success. Studies have confirmed that people who track their food intake are more likely to lose weight and maintain their weight loss. To track your intake properly, it will be best to write down everything you eat. You should include meals, snacks, and even the piece of candy you took from your co-worker's desk.

It is also advisable to record your emotions in your food journal. This will help you to identify certain overeating triggers and help you find healthier ways to manage them.

Celebrate Your Successes

Losing weight is not a walk in the park. Therefore, celebrate all your successes and use them to keep yourself motivated. Give yourself a pat on the back every time you accomplish a goal. For instance, social media and weight loss websites are ideal places to share your success and get support. Your motivation will increase as you develop pride in yourself.

You should also learn to celebrate behavior changes and not just certain numbers on the scale. For instance, if you met your goal of exercising four days a week, you can celebrate your achievement by planning a fun night with friends. You can increase your motivation by rewarding yourself for the habits.

But it will only help if you choose appropriate rewards. Don't reward yourself with food. It is not a must to go for expensive rewards that you might not be able to buy. And the reward should not be so insignificant that it doesn't bring about a feeling of satisfaction.

Examples of great rewards include:

- Enrolling in a cooking class.
- Going to a movie.
- Buying new running shoes.
- Going for a manicure.

Make a Commitment

According to studies, individuals who make a public commitment are more likely to follow through with their goals. In this regard, letting others know about your weight loss plans will help you stay accountable. Tell your family and friends about your goals, and share them on social media if you have a supportive community there that you participate in. The more people you share your goals with, the greater the accountability.

Also, if you invest in a gym membership, or pay upfront for exercise classes, you are more likely to follow through because you have already invested.

Don't Go for Perfection and Learn to Forgive Yourself

Remember, you don't have to be perfect to lose weight. If you approach weight loss with an all-or-nothing mindset, you are less likely to achieve your goals. Studies have revealed that individuals who are too restrictive usually find it challenging to stick to their diet plans.

Therefore, it is advisable to avoid being harsh with yourself whenever you make mistakes. Having self-defeating thoughts will dampen your motivation to continue. Instead, learn to forgive yourself, and remember that one mistake is not enough to mess up your progress.

Plan for Challenges and Setbacks

In your journey, you will encounter everyday stressors. You can plan ahead for these and develop the appropriate coping skills to help you stay motivated no matter the challenges you face. There will always be parties, holidays, and birthdays to attend. You will also encounter stressors at work or with family.

It is vital to start brainstorming about how you are going to deal with these possible setbacks. This ensures that you remain on course and stay motivated. For instance, many people turn to food whenever they are feeling stressed. This could easily lead them to discard their weight loss goals entirely for the instant gratification they receive from food.

If you create appropriate coping skills, you can avoid this happening to you.

According to studies, people who can handle stress better and have better coping strategies, usually lose more weight and keep it off for longer. Some stress-coping methods you can use include:

- Exercising
- Taking a bath
- Going out and to get some fresh air
- Asking for help
- Talking to a friend

DOES MOTIVATION FOR WEIGHT LOSS WORK?

Success Story: Jane Shaw

Jane had had an athletic body up until she got married. She stopped working out and rapidly gained over 100 pounds. In 2017, she reached her highest weight—340 pounds. Jane felt like a stranger in her own body. She didn't recognize the woman she saw in the mirror, and she felt disgusted.

For six years, she tried losing weight with fad diets and multiple weight loss programs. Unfortunately, none of them seemed to be working. She could no longer fit in her favorite dresses, and some of her friends and family made pointed comments about how she looked. She was devastated about this issue.

Her sister's wedding was fast approaching, and she was supposed to be one of the bridesmaids. This acted as a motivation for her to lose weight, and, at first, she considered getting gastric bypass surgery but had to lose some weight before she qualified for the procedure.

In the first two months following a new eating plan, she lost 55 pounds; and then by the fifth month, she had lost 100 pounds. It was at this point that she decided not to go for gastric bypass surgery. She took it to the next level by introducing exercising to her regimen. Initially, she started by just walking, but later joined a gym that she goes to five days a week and continues to walk on the weekends.

In her own words, she believed that she is stronger than she ever thought she could be. She claims that she never had the confidence before, but now she was proud of how far she had come. She can run, do burpees, push-ups, and planks.

She claims that celebrating small victories and the support from her husband and other family members were critical to her success. While recording her story, she was excited about her sister's wedding as she couldn't wait to wear a bridesmaid's dress that made her feel sexy.

As you can see, Jane's motivation to lose weight was extrinsic. The fact that she needed to fit in a certain dress pushed her to take drastic measures—gastric bypass surgery. And she having to lose some weight to go under the knife was yet another external motivator.

However, as she was getting ready for the surgery, she slowly developed intrinsic motivation. She started believing more in herself and began pushing herself for her own benefit. This has helped her to stay fit and make healthy living her everyday lifestyle.

KEY TAKEAWAYS

- There are two main types of weight loss motivation—extrinsic and intrinsic.
- Extrinsic motivation is essential to help you get started and help you achieve short-term goals.
- Intrinsic motivation is critical for long-term goals like reaching your desired weight and maintaining it.
- It is important to have a network of people who will support you throughout your journey.
- Setting small, realistic goals and rewarding yourself when you achieve them is an excellent way of staying motivated.

Up to this point, you have learned plenty of helpful tips for your weight loss journey. You have also read a lot about dieting and eating habits that do not work. To settle the issue of dieting and eating that does work once and for all, please flip over to the next chapter for a comprehensive discussion!

PART III

Normally, when you start a diet, you will lose weight right away, especially if you have the inspiration to get started and stick to your diet plan. However, in the long run, as you lose more weight your metabolism will slow down. And, like many other people, you will forget to adjust your other behaviors to match your new metabolism.

According to weight loss experts, as you lose weight, your metabolism will fight back against you and make it more challenging to remain on the downward trend. You need to be fully aware of what works best for you, and you need a plan that does not make you feel deprived, as this could lead you back to previous, unhealthy eating habits.

Diets can also harm you instead of help you. For example, a diet that encourages you to shun certain food types completely may leave you lacking certain essential nutrients. Additionally, the diet plans don't teach the consumers anything about healthy eating. As a result, once you are done with your diet plan, you will bounce back to the unhealthy eating habits that made you gain weight in the first place.

Studies examining the effectiveness of dieting also uncovered the fact that overly restrictive diets usually take some of the pleasure out of eating. They make losing weight sound and feel like a punishment, and there is a better way of doing things. Some other researchers have even found that dieting accompanied by frequent compulsive weighing is likely to lead you to eating disorders. People who diet are 8 times as likely to develop an eating disorder as those who don't.

Another thing that makes dieting ineffective is that most of the promoters are unscrupulous business people out to profit from other people's desperation to lose weight. If you have grappled with weight loss for some time, you may have become the prey of these crafty individuals and companies who claim to have a "magic weight loss potion." You may also notice that they claim that this magic potion works well if accompanied by healthy eating and regular physical exercise. But you can forget the magic potion entirely; it is the healthy eating and exercise that are actually at work!

Some people become obese because of an ordeal early on in life. The findings of this study showed that the majority of individuals with obesity had had various challenges when they were young. For such people, a dieting plan wouldn't help them. They need therapy sessions to help them address the problem at its roots.

DIFFERENT TYPES OF RESTRICTIVE OR UNSUSTAINABLE FAD DIETS

A fad diet promises users weight loss, or any other health advantages, without concrete scientific backing. The diets are also called popular diets or diet cults. Fad diets are

usually very restrictive, and in some cases, they require users to eliminate whole foods types like grains and dairy. The desired diet is often made up of expensive and superfluous food products and ingredients that are not nutritionally balanced and are ineffective in the long run.

Here are examples of the restrictive diets

Vegan or Vegetarian

Nutritionists argue that a vegan lifestyle based on a balanced diet can have many health benefits. But, most of the people who choose this diet are not necessarily including enough fruits and vegetables in their meals. They often eliminate major food groups, leading to deficiencies in protein, vitamins, and minerals. The notable elements missing in many vegan diets include iron, iodine, vitamin B12 and D, zinc, calcium, and proteins.

On the other hand, vegetarians are less at risk of nutrient deficiencies because some still take dairy, eggs, and fish. Nevertheless, it would be best if you eat well-balanced meals that contain all food groups.

Juice Cleanse

A juice cleanse usually lasts between a few days to several weeks. While you might experience weight loss during the juice cleanse, remember that it is just a temporary outcome.

Juice is rich in vitamins and minerals, but it is also full of sugar and deficient in fiber. Without fiber, protein, and other nutrients from food, the juice cleanse could make you feel lethargic and irritable. You could also experience irregular bowel movements and reduced productivity.

Ketogenic Diet

The ketogenic diet is usually very low in carbohydrates, with moderate protein and very high in fat. The diet has become very well known in recent years, thanks to celebrity endorsement. However, as you adopt this lifestyle, you will be eliminating a few important food groups from your diet.

Nutritional experts warn that any overly restrictive diet plan cannot be a long-term and sustainable healthy diet. However, it is important to note that there are individuals on a ketogenic diet for medical reasons. Such individuals are under strict supervision by their physicians, as it is usually used to control epilepsy and other long-term conditions.

Paleo Diet

We also know the paleo diet as the caveman diet. It goes back to the basics by focusing on natural foods instead of processed ones. However, its shortcomings include being heavy on meat and excluding other important food types like grains, dairy, and legumes, which have key roles to play in our bodies.

Gluten-Free

Gluten-free diets usually originate from medical necessity. Doctors normally advise individuals with celiac disease and gluten sensitivities to avoid gluten-rich foods to help them manage symptoms. If you don't suffer from any of the two cases, there is no scientific evidence suggesting that it could work as a weight loss option.

As mentioned earlier, fad diets are popular, and you will always see new plans attempting to solve people's need to lose weight fast. However, most of these fad diets are unbalanced and won't live up to your expectations. Additionally, the diet might work in the short term, but it is not sustainable in the long run. It will be best to find a healthy way of eating that you enjoy and will enable you to achieve and maintain your preferred weight.

EATING DISORDERS AND WEIGHT STIGMA

The word *eating* in the phrase *eating disorder* is usually misleading. You see, eating disorders are more than just food intake fixations. According to expert definitions, they are complex, mental-health conditions that normally require the intervention of medical and psychological experts to change their course. Studies have suggested that nearly 20 million women in the United States have had an eating disorder at some point in their lives.

FACTORS AFFECTING FOOD CHOICES

Several factors determine our food choices. In the current world, humans give dietary change a priority in achieving different objectives. However, it is critical to understand the determinants that influence our food choices. In this part, I will take you through the main influences on our food choice, focusing on the amenable ones and effective interventions.

What Are the Major Determinants of Food Choice?

You might be thinking, *the key driver for eating is hunger, duh!* You are right to a degree. Several studies have confirmed that whatever you choose to eat is not only determined by nutritional and physiological needs.

The factors that influence our food choice include:

- Biological determinants like taste, appetite, and hunger.
- Economic determinants like availability, cost, and income.
- Physical determinants like education, cooking skills, and access.

- Social determinants like family, culture, meal patterns, and peers.
- Psychological determinants like guilt, mood, and stress.
- Beliefs, knowledge, and attitudes.

As you can see, there is some level of complexity when it comes to food choice despite the list not being exhaustive. Moreover, the power of each determinant varies from one individual to the other. So the type of food intervention that works for you might not work for someone else. Let's look at each of the determinants in more depth.

Biological Determinants

Hunger and Satiety: Your psychological needs usually provide the primary determinants of food choice. The human body requires energy and nutrients to survive and it responds strongly to feelings of hunger and satiety. Your central nervous system controls the balance between hunger, food intake, and appetite stimulation.

Nutritionists state that different types of food generate varying satiety signals. According to research, fat has the lowest satiating effects, and low-density diets create greater satiety than high energy density diets.

Palatability: Palatability has all to do with the pleasure you experience when you eat a particular food. Palatability depends on the sensory properties of food like smell, taste, texture, and appearance. For example, sweet and high-fat foods usually have an incontestable sensory appeal.

As a result, food is not only considered a source of nourishment but also a source of enjoyment. Multiple studies have looked into the influence of palatability on food intake and appetite, and have confirmed that people tend to consume more when the food is palatable.

Sensory Aspects: Taste undoubtedly has a major influence on food-related behavior. It can be defined as the sum of all sensory stimulation that is generated when you ingest food. This also includes appearance, smell, and texture. Sensory aspects normally affect your spontaneous food choices.

From your childhood on, taste and familiarity affect your attitude toward food. It is also regarded as a natural human trait to like sweetness and dislike bitterness. As we grow, our expectations, beliefs, and attitudes influence our food preferences and dislikes.

Economic and Physical Determinants

Cost and Accessibility: The cost of food is another one of the primary determinants of food choice. Your income and socio-economic status determine whether the cost will be prohibitive. According to reports, low-income groups have a greater tendency to eat unbalanced diets. They are also reported to consume fewer vegetables and fruits. Nevertheless, access to more money does not automatically result in a better quality diet, but the range of foods from which you can choose will increase.

Another critical factor that affects our food choices is accessibility to shops. Accessibility depends on factors such as geographical location and transport. Healthy food tends to be more costly in towns and cities.

Education and Knowledge: Experts argue that a person's level of education usually affects their dietary behavior well into their adulthood. Conversely, having nutrition knowledge and having good dietary habits are not always related. Studies suggest that having knowledge on health does not lead to action if you don't know how to apply the knowledge.

Besides, people get information on nutrition from different sources, which can sometimes be conflicting or lack reliability. It is critical to read accurate information on nutrition from credible sources that have earned the right to influence your decisions.

Social Determinants

Social Class Influence: Your social and cultural practices will constrain what you eat. Many studies have shown that differences in social classes correlate with our food and nutrient intake. Poor diets usually result in nutritional deficiencies or obesity, which is a problem that different sectors of our society face.

Cultural Influence: Cultural influences shape your attitude towards certain foods. Things like the chronic consumption of certain foods and preparation traditions usually lead to restrictions like excluding meat or milk from your diet. Luckily, cultural influences are amenable to change. For example, when you move to a new country, you will adapt to the new food habits of the local culture.

Psychological Factors

Stress: Psychological stress has unfortunately become a common feature in modern society. Studies have also shown that this can modify several behaviors that affect your health. The different types of stress that humans experience make the influence of stress on food choices even more complex. Moreover, the effect of stress on food choice depends on the individual, the circumstances, and the stressor. For instance, some people eat more while others eat less when under pressure.

Mood: Studies have shown that food influences your mood, and it can also affect your food choice. It is also riveting to note that the influence of food on your mood is also closely related to your attitude toward certain foods.

EVIDENCE SUPPORTING THE ROLE OF THE MIND IN WEIGHT LOSS

Psychology is the study of why people do the things they do. There is enough evidence to suggest that the mind plays a critical role in your weight loss journey. Experts have revealed that your mind plays two key roles in weight loss:

- **Behavior** – Your therapist will help you identify habitual patterns of eating then help you learn how you can change them.
- **Thinking (cognition)** – For this, your therapist focuses on discovering self-defeating patterns that contribute to issues with weight management.

How the Mind Helps in Weight Management

Many weight loss experts use cognitive-behavioral treatment because it addresses your thinking patterns and behavior. The treatment covers the following areas.

Determines your readiness to change. This entails an awareness of what you need to do in order to achieve your goals. It also involves committing to the plan you've made for yourself.

Teaches you how to monitor yourself. Self-monitoring helps you to be more conscious of what triggers you to eat. It also makes you more mindful of your food choices and portions. Self-monitoring can help you to remain focused on your long-term goals.

Shows you how to break unbeneficial patterns. Your therapist will use stimulus control to teach you how to break any links between eating and other activities. For instance, you stop eating in certain settings and avoid displaying poor food choices in your kitchen.

Helps you find healthy distractions. This therapy helps you replace eating with healthier outlets. Other techniques used include positive reinforcement, problem solving, social support, and the change of eating habits.

Weight loss therapists and coaches discovered the importance of the mind in the entire process. As a result, most weight loss programs incorporate cognitive therapy sessions to help address how you think about food. The therapy also helps you identify self-defeating patterns of thinking that usually undermine the success of any weight loss endeavor. It helps the subjects learn and practice using positive coping self-statements.

The bottom line is that you must change your thinking if you want to lose weight. Studies have confirmed that you must change your lifestyle if you want to manage your weight. It is also apparent that those who depend on diet programs to lose weight usually fail in their attempts.

To succeed, you must realize the role eating plays in your life. It would be helpful if you also learned how to use positive thinking and other behavioral coping approaches to manage your eating and weight.

GOLDEN RULES OF EATING

As you look for the best formula to lose weight, you might find yourself caught up in the world of dieting. As you look for the next program to help you, you should consider your health the number one priority. Most of the dieting programs don't focus on helping you set up a healthy future.

Here are the golden rules of eating to keep your health in the spotlight:

Don't Starve Yourself

The first golden rule of eating is not starving yourself. If your diet plan forces you to stay hungry for up to 24 hours, you need to look for a new plan. Such a diet does not contain all the right foods to promote satiety and does not offer enough calories to help you sustain yourself. The truth is, starvation diets don't work; the sooner you come to terms with this, the better.

Eat Multiple Food Groups Daily

Healthy eating also involves eating well-balanced foods every day. You should avoid any diet plans that encourage you to leave out certain food groups from your diet. For example, some diets advise users to shun grains completely. Well, even if you are gluten-free, ensure that you are eating a diet containing sources of complex carbohydrates. You can try sweet potatoes, bananas, or beans.

Nutritionists advise that your daily diet should contain a balanced mix of nutrients. Particularly, your meals should have healthy fats, lean proteins, and carbohydrates, including both the high-starch and high-fiber varieties.

Limit Artificially Prepared Foods

The other golden rule of healthy eating is avoiding artificially prepared foods. In short, if a food is formed by man, then it is preferably not something you should be ingesting. It is best to eat foods that are in their most natural state.

Popular examples include fruits, nuts, vegetables, and seeds. Such food will give you a higher amount of nutrition and help you fuel your body for your daily activities. On the other hand, manufactured foods generally pop out and leave you feeling fatigued.

Don't Be Overly Restrictive

It is also helpful to avoid being too restrictive so your plan can be sustainable. An excellent, healthy, and sustainable eating plan should help you maintain a good relationship with food. For instance, go for a plan that allows you to eat that piece of cake occasionally and even go out with friends to enjoy your favorite restaurants.

It is critical to note that you should build your diet in moderation. Otherwise, if you become too restrictive and compulsive, you are likely to develop a bad relationship with food.

Here is a dietary routine for main meals that will support your healthy eating:

Food #1: Vegetables Low in Calories Take the Lead

According to the American Diabetes Association, fresh vegetables, greens, and garden produce are compulsory in putting together a healthy lunch or dinner. In this regard, consider having half of your plate filled with these kinds of foods. If you follow this rule, it will create a big shift from your usual eating dynamics with just one change.

For example, the biggest dilemma you normally experience when preparing a main meal is what kind of protein you will use and how you will present it. However, with this new thinking, the first thing you must consider is which non-starchy vegetables you will use and then plan your menu around that. It is also advisable to go for fresh produce instead of frozen or preserved.

Food #2: Whole Grain or Starch-Rich Cereals

After elaborating half your menu with low-starch foods, your next order of business is to take the remaining half of your plate and divide it into two quarters. Fill one of the two parts with a recipe based on ingredients rich in complex carbohydrates. Great examples to choose from include cereals, corn, and rice. You can also go for any other foods that are rich in starch.

Food #3: Healthy Sources of Protein

Use this food group to fill the remaining quarter of your plate. Go for protein sources such as lean meats, fish, and eggs. However, you should also consider including pulses, better known as legumes, in your meals. They are an unfairly forgotten element in many food menus, but include excellent sources of protein and fiber with a low-fat content.

HOW YOU CAN REWIRE YOUR BRAIN FOR A HEALTHY LIFESTYLE

By now, you are well aware that your brain plays an important role in your weight loss journey. For instance, experts suggest that the food you eat and how you consume it usually triggers a chemical response in your brain that can eventually block weight loss, creating insatiable hunger and overpowering cravings.

The most troublesome cravings are the ones for sugar and flour, which make up almost everything we consume. They can hijack your neurotransmitters and hormones, leading to changes to your brain that make you crave more of them. In short, they are very addictive!

However, if we make correct food choices, we can heal our brains and make them work for us and not against us, helping us achieve sustainable weight loss.

Here are five straightforward steps to rewire your brain:

Minimize Sugar and Flour

Flour and sugar have the same addicting effect on your brain as cocaine and other hard drugs. They are known for stimulating your brain's seat of motivation, reward, and pleasure. Eventually, they will lead you to increase the intake of them in order to experience the same level of bliss. That is a great example of addiction.

Moreover, flours and sugars usually block your brain from recognizing leptin, the hormone that sends the signal from your stomach to your brain that you are full. Without leptin, you will eat past the point of feeling full until your stomach hurts. The only way to get out of this vicious cycle is by detoxing your brain from flour and sugars.

Eat Regularly

You can train your brain to eat the right things at the right times by having a consistent schedule of three meals a day. This routine will also help you to pass up the wrong things you would have consumed in between sporadic meals because of sudden hunger.

Eat the Right Quantities

Many adults no longer get reliable signals from their brains to stop eating when they have eaten enough food. When

you eat the right portions, you revive these signals over time, and that only will help you melt the pounds off.

Consistency

Being consistent is the key to unlearning bad eating habits and learning better ones. Consistency takes the burden off your willpower, making good choices feel more natural. It also gets rid of the ambiguity that gives room for one more bite. When your brain is rewired, you will maintain your goal weight and achieve exercise milestones with less resistance.

SUCCESS STORY

Name: Gracie Barnes

Success Story: Gracie lost 106 pounds without going to the gym!

Gracie had gone through a lifetime of struggles as she attempted to lose weight. One unique approach she took that nearly got her killed was fad dieting. She bought a diet plan online that advised her to starve for hours to help her lose weight. However, her motivation to lose weight was her negative view of her body and her embarrassment.

While she did lose a few pounds, it actually felt like a punishment. After failing to achieve her target weight after several months of torturing herself, she became so depressed that she ended up in the hospital.

It is here that someone introduced her to a different way of approaching her goal. She stopped all the calorie counting and overly restrictive diets, and the new plan involved keeping things simple. She only ate when she felt hungry and stopped when she was full. She made it a point to go on a walk every day to remain active.

She also became very mindful of the things she eats, which helped her start making better food choices. Her meals are mainly fresh vegetables and fruits, but she also takes smaller portions of healthy carbohydrates and proteins.

After practicing her new routine, she has lost 106 pounds without stepping into the gym. The turning point was learning to love herself and make changes to her eating habits for her health and not the scale. She documented her journey on social media, where she was able to receive plenty of support from her followers and has also gotten many people requesting that she help them lose weight.

KEY TAKEAWAYS

- Fad diets usually sound very enticing, but they don't work in the long run! They might help you quickly shed some weight, but you are very likely to backslide.

- Most restrictive diets are used for medical cases under the strict supervision of a physician. Don't follow them blindly or without a doctor's recommendation.
- You should be aware of the factors that affect your food choices and make changes where you can. For instance, you can change your mind about certain cultural beliefs that stop you from consuming healthy foods.
- Eating has golden rules that work excellently in your weight loss journey. It shouldn't feel like a punishment.
- Your brain could let you down if you don't rewire it for weight loss and healthy eating success. You must align your brain with your journey by rewiring it for sustainable healthy living.

Toot your horn for coming this far. We are getting close to the end of our journey together. Have you chosen your favorite weight loss method yet? In the upcoming chapter, you will discover more about the principles of nutrition.

9

PRINCIPLES OF NUTRITION

*H*ave you ever heard the phrase, you are what you eat? Well, this phrase has become a point of truth in contemporary society. Agriculture, healthcare, and society at large are struggling with food, diet, and processing methods. There is a newfound awareness and concern with sustainable food production methods.

The science of nutrition is a somewhat modern subject. As a matter of fact, the role of nutrition in obesity and chronic diseases has only recently come to the fore. Nutrition is critical to all types of health, including physical and emotional health. Regrettably, it is not possible to out-train a bad diet, so it is necessary to learn the principles of nutrition.

The simple truth is that if you don't eat right, it is impossible to attain the body size you want. You will not have the confidence you deserve nor the health required to support a long and energetic life. The splendid news is that you don't have to continually suffer to reach your weight loss goals if you learn sustainable eating habits that are inspired by the core principles of nutrition.

For instance, I usually enjoy hamburgers and hot dogs. At the same time, I also eat a lot of salad and vegetables because I understand the principles of nutrition and how to use them effectively. It will be tremendously helpful to understand a few important variables that matter more than everything else combined. In this chapter, you will learn about proper nutrition and how a balanced diet affects your weight loss success. You will also learn the secret of accounting for social situations and special circumstances. When you combine the knowledge gained from the previous chapters with what you will learn here, your life won't remain the same again.

WHAT IS PROPER NUTRITION?

Simply put, good nutrition means that your body is getting all the nutrients, and minerals that it requires to work at its best. Unfortunately, most people complicate the issue of proper nutrition, but the core principles of nutrition are straightforward and learnable.

The human body requires six classes of nutrients—classified as substances—for nourishment, growth, and development. They are essential to life and include:

- Water
- Carbohydrates
- Fats and fatty acids
- Minerals
- Vitamins
- Proteins

These nutrient classes are broken down into two main categories: micronutrients and macronutrients. Macronutrients include carbohydrates, proteins, and fats, which give your body the energy it requires to work well and work for you.

On the other hand, micronutrients don't provide energy but are critical to other body processes and overall health. They include minerals and vitamins that you consume in smaller quantities.

WHY THESE NUTRIENTS ARE CRITICAL

You must incorporate the basic principles of nutrition into your daily diet and lifestyle habits. It is also preferable to apply these principles in the form of unprocessed foods. Whenever you add sugar or artificial colors and flavors to your food, you alter its texture and stability. That food will then be classified as processed.

Studies have linked heavily processed foods to higher risks of obesity, high blood pressure, and cholesterol levels.

WHERE CAN YOU FIND THESE CRITICAL NUTRIENTS?

Water

Scientists have confirmed that the adult human body is made up of 60% water. Therefore, keeping yourself hydrated is critical for survival. The amount of fluid needed in a human body depends on various issues, including age, climatic conditions, levels of physical activity, and diet.

You should eat foods with a high water content and drink plenty of water to help your body:

- Lubricate your joints and eyes.
- Get rid of waste.
- Regulate temperature.
- Reach a point of general health and wellness.

Carbohydrates

Carbohydrates are essential nutrients that many people often misunderstand and view in a negative light. Your body needs carbohydrates for optimal energy, and as one of the macronutrients, you can find most carbs in plant-based foods like grains, legumes, beans, fruits, and vegetables.

Carbohydrates are undoubtedly the primary and preferred source of energy for your body, and they can protect you from disease. For instance, there is evidence showing the importance of whole-grain foods and dietary fiber from whole foods in reducing the risk of cardiovascular disease. Fiber also protects you against obesity, type 2 diabetes, and is also essential for your digestive health.

There are two main kinds of carbohydrates, i.e. sugars and starches, and both provide your body with the energy it needs. Sugars are also subdivided into:

- Intrinsic – These are sugars that are part of the cellular structure of foods. For example, fruits and vegetables contain intrinsic sugars.
- Extrinsic – These are not part of the cellular structure of foods. Examples of this include lactose contained in dairy products, honey, confectionery, and fruit juices.

Complex carbohydrates comprise starch and non-starch polysaccharides. You can get starch from potatoes, bread, pasta, and rice, while non-starch polysaccharides are contained in vegetables, fruits, whole grain cereals, and legumes.

Fiber is a type of carbohydrate that you mainly get from plant-based foods. Because fiber is not digestible, it does not provide your body with energy. Nevertheless, it is essential for a healthy digestive system.

Half the energy in your diet should come from carbohydrates, especially starchy carbohydrates. Beware that if you frequently consume foods and drinks containing non-milk extrinsic sugars, you will risk tooth decay.

Proteins

Proteins comprise small building blocks referred to as amino acids, which are critical to creating new muscles, hormones, and enzymes. You can get your protein intake from animal and plant cells from several foods—including meat, fish, dairy, eggs, pulses, nuts, and cereals.

There are approximately 20 distinct amino acids in foods. The amino acids can be broken down into two main groups:

- **Essential Amino Acids** – These are the ones that your diet must supply. They include isoleucine,

leucine, threonine, valine, methionine, lysine, tryptophan, and phenylalanine. Also, children need plenty of histidine because their bodies cannot produce enough to meet their needs.

- **Non-Essential Amino Acids** – These are the amino acids that the human body can make itself. It does this by breaking down the amino acids in protein that you consume and absorbs them to form other proteins.

Different types of foods supply your body with different amounts and combinations of amino acids. Suppose you are a vegan or vegetarian, you can get all of your proteins by combining different plant-based sources of protein.

Fats

Fats have a bad reputation. Nevertheless, they are critical in helping you maintain your blood sugar level, balancing your hormones. and enhancing your overall brain function. Moreover, they can also help you to lower your risk of heart disease and type 2 diabetes. Fat also acts as an anti-inflammatory, which helps to lower the risk of cancer, arthritis, and Alzheimer's disease. They are also critical in helping your body to absorb fat-soluble vitamins like A, D, E, and K.

You can get the fat your body needs from meat, meat products, fish, eggs, dairy products, nuts, cereals, vegetables, fruits, and cereal products like biscuits and cakes. Fats can either be saturated or unsaturated depending on the fatty acids they contain. For instance, butter is described as a saturated fat because it contains more saturated fatty acids than unsaturated fatty acids. On the other hand, olive oil is regarded as unsaturated fat because it contains more unsaturated fatty acids than saturated fatty acids.

You can source saturated fats from animal products, while we get our unsaturated fats from vegetable sources. But there are several exceptions. You can convert unsaturated fats into saturated fats through a process known as hydrogenation.

You must supply essential fatty acids (EFAs) in your diet because your body cannot make them. There are two essential fatty acids:

- Alpha linolenic acid (n-3)
- Linolenic acid (n-6)

Your body uses these two essential fatty acids to synthesize other fatty acids. Fat should not be more than one-third of your energy intake. Moreover, a high intake of saturated fat can have undesirable effects on your health.

Vitamins

Vitamins are one of the necessary micronutrients. They are organic compounds that contain carbon and are naturally sourced through a diverse and healthy diet. The essential vitamins include:

- Vitamin A – Critical for your skin and eyes.
- Vitamin B – Building blocks for your body's health. It helps you maintain energy levels, cell metabolism, and brain function.
- Vitamin C – Essential for your bone and muscle structure and immune system.
- Vitamin D – Necessary for bone growth, as well as nervous and cardiovascular health.
- Vitamin E – Protects against cell damage.

Vitamins A, C, D, and E are known as antioxidants. Other vitamins essential to your body include B1, B2, niacin, B6, B12, and folate of water-soluble vitamins. Because your body cannot make them, you must supply yourself with all vita-mins except vitamin D. For vitamin D specifically, your body can produce it through the exposure of sunlight on your skin. The amount of vitamins your body requires changes throughout your lifetime.

Minerals

Minerals are the other chemical elements that your body needs apart from hydrogen, carbon, nitrogen, and oxygen. You can find these nutrients in a well-balanced diet. They are essential for bone and teeth formation and are also an essential component of your body's fluids and tissues. You also need minerals for proper nerve function and enzyme productions.

Different foods provide different amounts of minerals. The minerals essential to your body include iron, zinc, magnesium, calcium, sodium, phosphorus, chromium, potassium, iodine, selenium, fluoride, copper, and chloride. Your body needs a different amount of each of these minerals for various processes, and there are some minerals that your body requires in large amounts. For example, phosphorus, calcium, chloride, potassium, magnesium, and sodium are all in this category.

Now that you know the critical nutrients that your body needs, it's time to look at the five principles of nutrition to live by.

PRINCIPLES OF NUTRITION TO LIVE BY

Even though nutrition is often confusing, uncertain, and debated passionately, the principles you will learn here are undeniable and transformative. Research has shown that experts agree on these five nutrition principles that are supported by scientific evidence. These are the nutrition concepts that you can rely on.

1. The Principle of Energy Balance

This is the energy balance equation that everyone knows about, but not everyone believes in. It is also referred to as calories in, calories out (CICO), and is usually represented like this:

[Energy in] – [Energy out] = Changes in Your Body

This means that you will gain weight when you ingest more energy (calories) than you burn. On the other hand, when the energy you ingest is less than the amount you burn, you will lose weight. Finally, when the energy you ingest is equal to the energy you burn, you will maintain the same weight. Simple, right?

I know you are wondering, how do I know this with utter sureness? Well, this principle is straightforward to confirm. If you reduce the energy that goes into your body and increases the energy you burn, you will lose weight. This principle is based on the first law of thermodynamics—energy is neither created nor destroyed; you can only transfer it from one state to another. In this regard, human beings cannot create energy from nothing. They simply convert it from food. Therefore, any excess energy you take in does not vanish magically. Your body will either increase energy put out by increasing metabolism or store the excess energy as fat.

To avoid falling into the confusion brought on by people who argue that not all calories are equal, let's look at the complex factors that influence calories in and calories out. For instance, your brain can either turn up or turn down your metabolism, thereby significantly influencing the calories out.

Here is the energy balance table:

Factors Influencing Energy In	Factors Influencing Energy Out
Your appetite. This is affected by hormones that regulate appetite and satiety.	The energy you burn as you rest. This is determined by your body size, hormonal status, genetic factors, dieting history, age, quality of sleep, and health status.
The food you consume. This is affected by availability, education, culture, palatability, socioeconomic status, sleep quality, and energy density.	The energy you burn through exercise. This is affected by your ability to exercise, frequency, duration, intensity, environment, type, sleep quality, and hormonal status.
The calories absorbed. This is influenced by food preparation, age, macronutrient intake, energy status, health status, and personal microbiome.	The energy you burn through non-exercise activities. This is influenced by factors such as genetics, energy status, health status, leisure activities, stress levels, occupation, and hormonal status.
Physiological factors such as mindset, stress levels, quality of sleep, perceived control, and self-esteem.	The energy you burn by metabolizing food. This is affected by the makeup of macronutrients and how processed your food is.

The law of gravity can also be referenced to help you understand energy balance. The basic law of gravity applies to any object that is dropped from any height. However, several other factors affect the basic principle, like air resistance, making the exact force downward vary even though the force of gravity is the same. The basic principle is constant; it applies to all foods you consume in all situations.

However, other factors affect parts of the equation and affect the result.

Therefore, if you want to lose weight, you must consider the overall energy balance and find ways to adjust it in your favor. Here are some secrets you can use to get started:

How to Reduce Calories In:

- Consume more proteins to reduce your appetite, which reduces your general energy intake.
- Eat slowly so that you can be attuned to your body's hunger and fullness signals. Stop eating whenever you feel satisfied.
- Use hand portions to help you determine how much you consume.
- Get enough sleep to reduce hunger and cravings for sweets.

How to Increase Calories out:

- Add cardio to your routine to enable you to burn more calories.
- Include strength training to enable you to build more muscle, enhance your metabolism, and burn more calories.
- Increase your daily activity by using the stairs and

parking farther from your destination. You can also use an activity tracker like a mobile app to push you to take more steps.

- Boost your protein intake to increase the thermic effect of digestion.
- Practice self-care to help reduce stress and improve sleep. The two are critical for a healthy metabolism.

2. Get Enough Protein

There are two reasons why you should get your proteins right:

It will help you consume less without feeling hungry. Studies have revealed that proteins help people feel full for longer periods, which reduces intake and limits snacking. This is partly because proteins usually take longer to break down than fats and carbs. Moreover, proteins stimulate the release of satiety hormones in your gut.

As a result, when you eat more proteins, you usually eat less food. This usually makes a massive difference. For instance, if you double your protein intake, you will end up taking in 400 fewer calories each day.

Proteins make it easy for your body to build and maintain muscle. Your body cannot function well without sufficient proteins because it requires amino acids to generate essential molecules like hormones, enzymes, antibodies, and neurotransmitters. Therefore, when you don't consume enough proteins, your body plunders them from other sources, like your muscles, leading to muscle loss.

On the other hand, when you consume high-protein diets, it maximizes muscle protein synthesis, leading to more muscle gain. Your age, gender, and goals will determine the amount of protein you should consume each day.

3. Food Processing Reduces Nutrient Density

Take minimally processed whole foods like grains, nuts, eggs, and fish. You will enjoy their vast selection of nutrients such as minerals, vitamins, phytonutrients (plant nutrients), and zoonutrients (animal nutrients). Several studies have revealed that you will be healthier if you consume more whole foods and less refined foods.

There is a well-known phrase, which states that "as food processing increases, nutrient density decreases." This is because the more processed food is, it loses nutritional value, including fiber, essential fatty acids, minerals, zoonutrients, phytonutrients, and vitamins. Additionally, processed foods have additives such as fillers, preservatives, sodium, sugar, unrefined starch, and unhealthy fats.

For instance, if you take a burger with fries, you consume 918 calories with 1012mg of sodium. On the other hand, a plate containing 6-ounce tenderloin, medium baked potato, and 2 cups of steamed broccoli has 562 calories and 108mg sodium.

From this comparison, you can see that whole foods are healthier than their more refined counterparts. As a result, it is sensible to eat diets rich in whole foods that are minimally processed. By doing this, you will avoid diseases such as cancer, depression, heart disease, and type 2 diabetes.

Moreover, minimally processed whole foods are rich in fiber and protein, which usually boost satiety. They also contain fewer calories per serving than highly processed foods. These traits are essential for weight loss.

Remember, the focus is not on perfection but rather progress. Your focus should be to make things a little better.

4. Fruits and Vegetables Are Your Best Friends

Studies have confirmed that fruits and vegetables can help you reduce the risk of getting sick and play a significant role in weight loss. Fruits and vegetables are rich in essential nutrients such as phytonutrients, fiber, vitamins, antioxidants, and minerals. These nutrients help your body avoid diseases such as cancer, blood pressure, stroke, and heart disease.

Besides, eating habits rich in these two can help you lose and control your weight. This is primarily because fruits and vegetables contain plenty of fiber and water, which helps to fill you up with fewer calories.

One golden nugget is to avoid sticking to one "magic power food." Instead, aim to eat a variety of fruits and vegetables. You can make it a habit to try and eat a wide rainbow of colors every day.

5. Sleep is Critical

In case you didn't know, sleep affects what you eat and your general wellbeing. According to studies, many people usually get everything right with their nutrition yet fail to reach their goals. Do you know why? They don't sleep enough! The studies also confirm that these individuals registered better results when they started to prioritize sleep.

What's the connection? You may ask. Well, if you sleep for 5 hours when your body needs 8 hours of sleep, your body remains in a chronic state of sleep deprivation. Consequently, this impairs your body's ability to regulate several critical hormones. Then this is what will happen:

- Your ghrelin levels go up hence triggering hunger.
- Your leptin levels fall, so you will take longer to feel full.

- Also, your endocannabinoids levels increase, making your perception of foods appear more gratifying.

All these effects make it challenging for you to keep away from the cookie jar! When you don't get enough sleep, these are the results:

- You are hungrier; hence you crave sweets more than you would.
- You feel tired, so you will not exercise, and you will reduce your movement.
- Furthermore, the more awake you are, the more time you have to raid your kitchen!
- Studies also reveal that one night of sleep deprivation can lead to an increase in your blood pressure the next day.

If you want a happy ending in your weight loss journey without interfering with your health, get enough sleep.

Golden Nugget: Ability to Regulate Your Internal Appetite is a Game-Changer

Many people depend on counting calories to guide them on how much they consume. While that can be helpful, it usually has its downside. As you follow strict macros and calorie counts, you essentially lose touch with internal cues that guide you on when to eat and when to stop. Therefore, stop thinking that having a strict food tracking system can help you reach your goals.

Instead, focus on learning to listen and respond to the internal sense of hunger and satiety. This is what is referred to as internal appetite regulation. As you relax and eat slowly, and tune into your thoughts, emotions, and bodily sensations, you make exceptional progress in regulating your appetite.

HOW TO ACCOUNT FOR SOCIAL SITUATIONS AND SPECIAL CIRCUMSTANCES

It is usually challenging for many people to have a normal social life when losing weight. Make no mistake; peer pressure is as real as it gets. Moreover, numerous temptations can overpower your willpower.

However, studies have revealed that you must continue with your social life even as you work on your weight loss program. Some experts argue that if you lose weight by exclusively eating from home, you are setting yourself up for failure once you finish the weight loss program. Therefore, you must learn to eat for the rest of your life in restaurants, at home, and in social situations.

When you go out, you get a perfect opportunity to test your new strategy of dealing with temptations. Moreover, gathering together with family and friends has legitimate psychological benefits. Social support is a critical element, especially when trying to achieve certain goals, including health and fitness goals. However, this does not mean that you RSVP yeas to all social events you are invited to.

You ought to be strategic in your approach to make choices that support your objectives. Examine every social opportunity to check whether it is suitable. Here are some guidelines to use:

- **Consider rare occasions.** It wouldn't be best to miss a wedding, graduation, or the chance to welcome a new baby into your family. Regardless of your fitness goals, you can use ways to stay on track and be part of these special occasions that come once in a while.
- **Consider the event's attendees**. Are they supportive of your goals? It is better to avoid events whose attendees don't value your health and fitness choices.
- **Consider how you will feel after the event.**

morning, please inform your friends that you will leave early because of the early morning run.

- **Have a snack before going to the party.** If you cannot bring a dish or the restaurant has not been selected beforehand, eat a filling snack. This will prevent you from making decisions inspired by extreme hunger.

- **Just say you are not drinking.** If you don't feel like drinking, just let your friends know and go for a club soda instead. You can even volunteer yourself as the designated driver.

- **Never give in to peer pressure**. Remember, no one can compel you to do what you don't want to do. As much as temptations and triggers exist, there is also pressure from friends, events, and places. However, always remember that you always have a choice, and you are entitled to do everything within your power to feel how you want to feel. This will help you make the best decision at every juncture.

HOW DO THE PRINCIPLES OF NUTRITION WORK IN WEIGHT LOSS?

Case Study: Cynthia – Lost Weight After Childbirth

When Cynthia got pregnant with her second child, she had some challenging times and turned to food to soothe herself. In the process, she gained a lot of weight - 100 pounds. In her own words – she self-medicated using food.

After giving birth, she made up her mind that she would use sustainable methods to lose weight. To her, that meant that she wouldn't deprive herself of any food group. Instead, she focused on eating until she was satisfied and practiced mindful eating to avoid stuffing herself.

Cynthia stated that her meals contained mainly lean protein, carbs, vegetables, and healthy fats. Moreover, she also changed her view of food. She stopped looking at food as a source of pleasure and started seeing it as a fuel source for her body.

After three months, she has lost 40 pounds, and her energy levels and stamina increased. In the 8th month of her weight loss journey, she had lost 100 pounds. Her advice to other women looking to lose weight is to create vision boards of where they want to be and what they want to look at.

Her vision boards contained goal-oriented images such as the outfits she aspired to wear, a healthy family, and the beach vacations she wanted to take. She stated that, as she looked on the vision boards every day, she could train her brain to herself as that fit, healthy person.

KEY TAKEAWAYS

- The human body requires all six classes of nutrients for nourishment, life and growth, and development. Therefore, your weight loss program should not deny you any of these classes of nutrients. You only need to know how to balance them.
- The principle of energy balance is the secret key. If you can learn how to balance "energy in" and "energy out", it becomes effortless to lose and maintain a certain weight.
- The more processed your food, the fewer nutrients it contains. Therefore, consider eating more minimally processed foods.
- You can still have a social life even when on a weight loss program. You only need to be disciplined enough to make the right choices.

Having read all the chapters to this point, you have all it takes to successfully lose weight without compromising your health. In the next chapter, I will let you in on how you can keep track of your progress.

10

TRACKING YOUR PROGRESS

*I*f you want your weight loss journey to be successful, this chapter is a must-read. Tracking your progress is a critical aspect of your weight loss endeavor. Unfortunately, many people are usually obsessed with the scale as a means of checking whether they are on the right track. Well, one thing you should be aware of is that the scale is the worst choice for tracking progress. As you will realize later in this chapter, your weight should be the least important thing you should be concerned about.

You must be thinking, is that right? Hold your horses and keep reading this chapter to understand what I mean. Here, you will learn how to truly keep track of your progress and the things you should focus on. Moreover, you will discover how to prepare your mind for weight loss success and also how to prepare your home, especially your kitchen, to ensure you succeed.

Another key thing you will learn in this chapter is how to manage your expectations. If you cannot manage your expectations, you might lack the motivation to keep going. At the end of this expertly crafted chapter, you will be well equipped to track your weight loss journey. So let's dive right in!

STOP OBSESSING WITH THE SCALE

It may sound preposterous, but the scale is not your best friend when keeping track of your weight loss. In fact, many experts argue that it is better at helping you maintain weight than it is at helping you when you are trying to lose weight.

This is a tough gospel, but multiple critical changes occur in your body that the scale cannot capture. Examples of these changes include:

- **The transformation happening inside.** You may not be aware of the changes that are happening in your cells when you exercise. However, what is happening behind the scenes can help you lose weight. When you exercise, you teach your body how to release more fat-burning

molecules. As your body becomes fitter, it burns more fat, and the scale might not capture that.

- **Changing body composition.** Although your weight is important, how much muscle you have is even more important. Muscle usually occupies less space than fat hence makes you look slimmer. Moreover, muscles are also more active metabolically. As you exercise, you gain more muscle, increase your metabolism and lose fat. Many times, these changes might not be captured on the weighing scale.

- **Strength and endurance.** If you exercise on a regular basis, you will be able to do more every time. When you start, you might exercise for a few minutes, but your body adapts gradually over time, allowing you to exercise for longer. This strength and endurance mean you are making some progress. However, if this is not showing on the scale, you might not realize how fit you are becoming.

There are several reasons why the weighing scale might not give you an accurate picture of your progress. One key reason is weight fluctuation; this will make the numbers on the scale fluctuate. When you see this happening, don't enter panic mode, it happens all the time.

So, why does your weight fluctuate? Here are some top factors to consider:

- **Muscle gain:** As you exercise, you lose fat and gain muscle, which takes up less space than fat. Muscle is heavier than fat and occupies less space. Therefore, you might be slimming down, but the scale's numbers tell a different story.

- **Food weight gain:** It might not be an excellent idea to weigh yourself after a meal. Food usually adds weight, so when you eat, your body will also add that weight. Luckily, this does not mean you have gained weight. It simply means you have added something to your body.

- **Water weight gain:** The human body is about 60% water. In this regard, fluctuations in your hydration levels can affect the number on your weighing scale. For instance, if you are dehydrated or have consumed a lot of salt, your body might retain water. In such a case, when you weigh yourself, the numbers on the scale might go up.

TRACK YOUR BODY FAT

Knowing your body fat percentage is critical to tracking your weight loss progress. This percentage is essential

because the scale weight does not tell the entire story. Once you know this percentage, you will have an idea of the amount of fat you need to lose.

It is possible to lose body fat and not lose weight. Therefore, if you are obsessed with the number on the scale, you might not notice you are slimming down. There are many alternatives for you to use to test your body fat, including:

- Online calculators
- Dual-energy X-ray absorptiometry (DXA scan)
- Calipers
- Bioelectrical impedance scales
- Hydrostatic weighing

How to get the most out of body fat measurement

- Check it weekly. You might not lose body fat overnight. Therefore, it would not be sensible to measure your body fat every day. In this regard, if you measure it daily, you might not see the small changes.
- Let one person measure your body fat. It is wise to stick with the same trainer to measure you. The reason is that different trainers use different methods so you might get different results.

- Have a journal. Track your numbers in a journal for accountability.
- Measure under the same conditions. If you are using the bioelectrical impedance scale, please make sure you measure under similar conditions. Things like food intake, hydration, and skin temperature can affect your body fat measurements.

TAKE BODY MEASUREMENTS

Apart from tracking your body fat, taking your body measurements is another excellent way of tracking your progress. Luckily, you don't need sophisticated equipment or a specialist to take them. Instead, experts argue that you can take measurements of certain areas of your body to help you discover where you are losing fat. This is critical because your body loses fat in different areas differently.

Taking these measurements will help you have the assurance that something is happening. You can start by wearing tight-fitting clothing then take notes. For instance, you can put on a swimsuit and take a picture. Then, the next time you measure yourself, put on the same swimsuit and take a picture. It would surprise you how much you can learn by looking at your pictures. Finally, you can wear the same clothing the next time you want to measure yourself to find out how tight they feel.

SUMMARY: HOW YOU CAN TRACK YOUR WEIGHT LOSS PROGRESS

Measure

Here are the parts you must measure:

- Bust
- Chest (under your bust)
- Forearm
- Thighs
- Upper arm
- Calves
- Waist

Measuring these body parts will give you a better picture of your body's composition. They will also help you understand why your scale numbers are not going down. Therefore, get yourself a tape measure and take these measurements at certain intervals.

Keep track of your workouts

Once you develop a regular workout routine and track your gym sessions, you should track all your sessions. You will literally see your wellness progress in your journal or workout app. For instance, if you could only do 15 push-ups the previous week and you can now do 25 in a row, that's progress! Of course, this applies to all the other exercises you do in your weight loss program.

How is your sex drive?

Several things affect your sex drive, including your workout, sleep quality, and the number of veggies you consume. So experts suggest that feeling a little bit randy is an excellent thing! Moreover, they argue that it shows you the other pieces of your health are in place. You can even get an app to help you track your sex drive.

Do you have a sleep App?

Health experts argue that good quality sleep is essential for recovery after your gym session. Moreover, lack of enough sleep usually increases your body's inflammation levels, contributing to the development of heart disease and Type 2 diabetes. Many fitness apps come with a sleep-tracking feature.

Have a journal

Studies have confirmed that individuals who spend some time alone usually improve their stress levels, find balance, and live healthier lives. Therefore, you should take some time at the end of each day to write down at least three things that made you feel good in your body.

Include the "big" and "small" things. As you take note of how you care for yourself every day, you will ensure your health, sanity, and wellness are on course.

How is your blood pressure?

It might not be the most popular way to record your progress but your blood pressure helps you track your heart health. For example, if there are no changes on the weighing scale numbers, your blood pressure can show you whether your risk for cardiovascular disease has decreased. It will also provide a concise picture of your overall health as other factors affect it, such as stress levels, nutrition, and exercise. Thanks to technology, you can find a mobile app for tracking your blood pressure on the go.

Keep track of your daily wellness goals

As you begin your days, please jot down at least three healthy goals you want to achieve in the next 12 hours. For instance, you can aim for five servings of fruits and veggies or walk 10000 steps. Then, later in the day, review your goals and check whether you achieved them all. Suppose you are achieving more goals on your to-do list; that's a sign you are getting healthier.

PREPARING FOR SUCCESS

When you read advertisements about weight loss diets that claim they have the magic bullet for your weight loss aspirations, you might think it will work like magic! Let me burst your bubble; that's a fallacy. The wise will tell you that chance will favor the prepared mind. Therefore, if you want to succeed in your weight loss journey, you have to prepare for it.

As we have already established in the previous chapters, your mind is where you win the weight loss battle. So, you have to have the right mentality if you want to sustain your weight loss program. Let's look at how you prepare your mind for weight loss success.

HOW TO PREPARE YOUR MIND FOR SUCCESS

Weight loss experts have confirmed that you need to have a mental makeover before you embark on your weight loss journey to help you overcome bad habits. The secret to beginning your transformation is having the right mindset. It is more sustainable to have a lifestyle change rather than going for a fad diet. You need to begin the journey aiming for weight control and remember that you want to maintain your new healthy diet.

Here are essential tips on how you can prepare properly for your weight loss journey:

Have clear weight loss goals

When you start with clear goals of what you want to achieve, it will help you to have the right mindset. Your goals could be as simple as looking and feeling better or more specific health goals like reducing high blood pressure or lowering the risk of diabetes. Having these goals will help you build the motivation you need to make your weight loss journey more enjoyable.

Write down your weight loss meal plan

After deciding your weight loss plan, write down the steps you need to implement it. Create a meal plan at the beginning of every week. This plan will guide you when you go shopping for groceries, preparing meals, and eating out. It will also help you avoid unplanned indulgences.

Moreover, when you have a meal plan it will help you to go for the right foods. For instance, before you go to a restaurant for dinner with friends, you can check out their menu online. This will help you to plan what you will order to avoid temptation once you are at the restaurant.

Invest in a personal trainer

One essential component of your weight loss journey is physical exercise. Weight loss experts suggest that you might not achieve your goals if you don't blend your diet plan with physical exercise. In this regard, consider working with a trainer or join a free consultation through a gym.

The professionals will help you to plan an exercise routine that you will enjoy. Planning will also help to fit your training routine into your daily schedule. Ensure that at the beginning of every week, you have marked every workout session in your calendar. It is easier to stick to the plan if it is in black and white.

Get the services of a dietitian

If you want to lose weight for life, you need to make an appointment with a licensed dietitian. Although you can follow any diet plan and lose weight, it might be detrimental to your health. Therefore, you need to work with a professional dietitian to help you develop a weight loss program suitable for your lifestyle, medical conditions, and dietary needs.

Weight loss experts argue that many of their clients had fallen off the wagon because they went for a diet plan that does not suit them. This is why you need the services of a licensed dietitian. Moreover, a professional dietitian can also help you to get ready mentally for the journey ahead. If you have medical insurance, check whether they provide reimbursement for nutrition counseling.

Get ready to log your fitness activities and food

One of the greatest secrets of success in weight loss is to log your diet and exercise activities. You can use the common pen and paper or use an online tool or mobile app. Regardless of your preferred choice, you should promise yourself that you will religiously outline and track all aspects of your weight loss process.

If you faithfully record every bite you eat, you will likely discover a certain pattern and routine. This makes it possible for you to find solutions to some eating problems that have derailed your earlier efforts to lose weight.

Have a realistic timetable for your weight loss journey

Studies have shown that people who set realistic weight loss goals are more likely to achieve them. You should remember that you are creating a lifelong strategy, so ensure you make them attainable. Forget about notions such as losing 15 pounds in 15 days.

Experts argue that the best approach would be to target losing like 2 pounds weekly for a prolonged period. You should use the same strategy for your workout exercises also.

If you are just getting started, don't try to run a marathon; start small and increase the exercises as you progress.

Have self-belief

Even if you failed in your previous weight loss attempts, it does not mean that you will also fail this time around. Remember, you will make several mistakes along the way, like eating more than you should or missing some planned exercises. When this happens, it is critical to remain positive and keep going.

It will help to accept that the weight loss goals will take some time to accomplish. It is also essential to believe that you can go the distance one step at a time. For instance, when you lose 5 pounds, that is great for your health and will give you the impetus you need to go on and lose the next 5 pounds. Please note that weight loss will not happen in a straight line; therefore, if you eat more than you should in one day, don't beat yourself up, get back on track and keep going.

Choose motivating rewards

Once you break your weight loss goals into achievable milestones, decide on the motivating rewards you will give yourself for reaching each milestone. As you choose your rewards, please don't go back to old patterns by going for a food reward. Alternatively, it is advisable to choose other types of treats like getting a massage, manicure, or going to a concert. You should also write down your rewards as part of your master plan.

Form a weight loss support network

Just like other life activities, your weight loss journey becomes easier when you surround yourself with a support system. Experts advise that you should have a weight loss network comprising your family members and friends. Moreover, they warn against announcing it to the whole world. Instead, just confide in your closest friends and family members.

Reveal to your network why you want to eat healthily and how they can support you to achieve your goals. It will be even better if you have a friend who is also trying to lose weight. You can agree to text each other at critical times of the day to help each other stay on track.

HOW TO PREPARE YOUR KITCHEN FOR SUCCESS

Once your mind is ready, you need to ensure there are no distractions. Therefore, the next thing is to set up your house, particularly your kitchen, for weight loss success. Studies have revealed that what you see in your kitchen usually significantly impacts your food choices.

In this regard, if you want to lose weight, you must make healthy food choices easily accessible. On the other hand, ensure you keep all the diet derailers out of sight. Here are specific things you can do to implement this strategy successfully:

Stock your fruit bowl

Studies have shown that women who keep a bowl of fresh fruit around their kitchen are 13 pounds lighter than their counterparts who don't. Fruits are a low-calorie snack, and displaying them on your kitchen counter reminds you to eat them instead of going for something else that could derail your goals. Moreover, the fruits are less tempting than chocolate, so you are only likely to eat one if you are really hungry.

Organize your pantry and fridge for success

You would have to keep all the junky snacks out of your home altogether in an ideal situation. However, if others in the house would like to have treats around, you need a strategy. The advisable way would be to store them in a place they won't tempt you each time you open the pantry or cupboard. Whatever trick you choose to use, please ensure it out of sight.

On the other hand, place the nutritious stuff in the spotlight zone in your fridge and pantry. When you keep healthy staples on the front shelves, they are more accessible. Also, studies suggest that your eyes will focus more on the center shelves. Therefore, consider filling your fringe's center shelves with healthy food choices.

Use the right containers

There is a high likelihood that not everything in your fridge is healthy. Therefore, consider placing the healthy foods in clear containers and using opaque containers for foods that are not so healthy. Studies have confirmed that what you see is what you will want to eat. This means that if you keep healthy foods in your line of sight, you are likely to eat them more.

Declutter your kitchen

You should not only concentrate on your fridge and pantry. It is also advisable to ensure that you clear all the clutter in your kitchen. For instance, always put away dirty dishes in the dishwasher instead of leaving them around the kitchen. You should also not have papers and other random junk piles up on your kitchen counters and tables.

Environment and behavioral experts suggest that spending time in a tidy kitchen reduces your stress levels. But, on the flip side, a messy kitchen causes additional stress, which triggers overeating.

MANAGING AND SETTING EXPECTATIONS

To this point, you are equipped with sufficient knowledge on how to successfully plan, execute and keep track of your weight loss journey. However, it is critical to know how to manage your expectations well regarding the progress that you are likely to make.

Remember that progress varies between different people; therefore, don't put too much pressure on yourself by comparing your progress to others. It is also seminal to remember that you don't have complete control of your weight loss journey. For instance, you don't have total control over the amount of weight you lose, the rate at which you lose it, and the body parts you lose it from. In this regard, you ought to manage your expectations as part of your long-term success.

Nevertheless, don't despair because there are many other aspects of your weight loss journey that you can control. Here are tips you can implement to manage your expectations:

The weight you will lose

The majority of individuals usually begin their weight loss journey with a particular number in mind. However, they might not have a concrete reason why that number is very important or where they got it from.

It is best to remember that your health is far more important. So, if you try to force your body to lose more weight than it can realistically, it could be detrimental to your health. You also need to remember that other things like pregnancies and medication can affect how your body stores fats, and it could be in ways out of your control.

Therefore, start by setting a goal that feels achievable and does not undermine your health. The goal is to make it enjoyable and keep adjusting as you progress. This ensures that you succeed again and again hence have enough motivation to keep going.

The time it will take

If you read most weight loss notebooks and journals, you will find individuals have indicated they want to shed a particular amount of weight within a specific period. For example, they could be getting ready for a wedding or getting their body in shape for the next bathing suit season.

While such goals might sound good, it is also critical to ask yourself if you had a weight gain time frame! You see, weight gain typically happens after some time while you are busy doing other things. News flash – weight loss happens the same way. Don't get it twisted; I am not saying there is something wrong with losing weight fast if you are on a healthy diet.

However, it has proven to be counterproductive to give yourself a compressed timeline to lose weight. You can quickly give up if you have an approaching deadline and some weight left to lose. Allow yourself to rethink this and focus more on non-scale, health-oriented goals and victories that motivate you to keep going. Focus on things you can control.

Body shape

It is important to accept that your body shape is something beyond your control. Remember that fat storage patterns are based on genetics. This means that if your genealogy has wide hips, you may not succeed in trying to compel your body to have slender hips.

So refrain from focusing on aspects of your body that are beyond your control. Instead, focus on health and weight loss aspects you can control like nutrition, enjoyment, and other lifestyle habits like exercising.

Your diet

Contrary to the lies propagated by many weight loss diet merchants, you can still lose weight by eating a nutritionally balanced diet. Therefore, in your weight loss journey, your health should take precedence. Avoid diets that advise you to disregard certain essential nutrients from your diets. You might achieve short-term success, but you might not like the long-term effects. Moreover, don't punish yourself with hunger by skipping meals to lose weight.

It is also possible to lose weight as you enjoy the food you eat. For instance, whenever you miss the foods you enjoy eating, you can try low-calorie recipes to help take care of your appetite and make you feel special. Learn to recreate the foods you love like pizza, bread, or any other calorically dense dishes into low-calorie versions.

How you look and feel

Remember, the goal is to focus on what you can control. Therefore, instead of focusing on the weighing scale numbers and time frames, consider goals like adding the number of days you exercise in your weekly routine. When you have such goals, your weight loss will happen the same way your weight gain happened.

This helps you to continually feel good about yourself because you know that you will keep improving your health even as you lose weight.

CASE STUDY

Whitney – Lost stubborn belly fat by tracking her progress

Before Whitney sought the services of a fitness coach, she had struggled to make significant progress in her quest to lose belly fat. Whitney claims that she had religiously followed her diet plan and exercise routines, but she was not making any progress.

However, after a couple of sessions with her coach, she revised her nutrition and workout routine. He started writing down everything, including her measurements, food intake, and exercises. As a result, she was also able to change her overall objective from losing her belly fat to living a healthier, more enjoyable life.

After a while, she realized that the belly fat was gradually disappearing without stressing herself about it. She was able to keep improving her exercise routines and her food choices. When writing her latest successful milestone, her belly fat was gone, and she had gained the strong body she wanted.

She was also happy because of the fact that her weight loss routine did not bar her from continuing with her social life.

She was happy that she now has developed a new healthier lifestyle that will help her maintain her physique!

KEY TAKEAWAYS

- The weighing scale does not tell the whole story. There is a lot of change taking place if you know where to look.
- Losing fat is critical in your weight loss journey. However, your weighing scale might not capture that. Use other means to measure your fat loss.
- If you don't keep track of your weight loss, you might lack the motivation to keep going.
- Managing expectations also ensures that you don't stress yourself over things you cannot control. It helps you to focus on achievable goals hence giving you the motivation you need for sustainability.

CONCLUSION

I will conclude this interesting read with a testimony from one of my clients. For privacy reasons, I will not disclose her true identity. For purposes of this section, we will call her Trina.

Trina started a blog post to record her weight loss journey, and I will share excerpts from her blog to demonstrate how hypnosis for weight loss works.

In her opening statement, she declared that

"I sought the help of a hypnotherapist because I desired to lose weight. However, I ended up learning something much deeper about myself that I didn't know!"

She further stated that her testimony was not a weight loss story but rather about how she found the path to the healthiest and happiest version of herself.

Trina reveals that she has had unhealthy eating habits since her college. She misused the freedom she had outside her parent's house to eat whatever she desired. The bad eating habits she developed in college got worse with time and became like an obsession. She reveals that she used to feel warm and happy, and comforted while eating. However, because she overdid it, she ended up feeling guilty and ashamed of herself.

Her obsession with food became a backdrop of her life as she continued with her life normally. She would engage in healthy eating and exercise for a week or two and then revert to her usual ways. But, unfortunately, she couldn't sustain a healthy lifestyle for long.

When she got married, things got worse. The first years in marriage were difficult, and she turned to food for comfort. This resulted in rapid weight gain, decreased energy levels. To make matters worse, she slid into depression.

After hitting rock bottom, she needed a helping hand to climb out of the hell hole she was in. she went to a doctor who prescribed for her a diet medication that promised results in glorified speed. It seemed to work as it curbed her appetite and gave her energy to exercise more actively than her body could in the past. She even claims that she started feeling "happier." In five months, she had lost 40 pounds.

Sadly, she couldn't continue using the pill forever as it had terrifying risks. As a result, she gained back 20 pounds after finishing the prescription. To stop her ballooning weight, she decided to starve herself. She came up with fasting days, but she suffered a lack of energy. With her new "punishing" routine, she could lose one pound or two every day and end up gaining 3 to 4 pounds during the weekends. She was accomplishing nothing and growing miserable by the day!

Then she was introduced to hypnotherapy.

She had heard about hypnotherapy for weight loss before, but like everyone else, she remained skeptical. However, with nowhere to run she contacted me. We had a conversation over the phone and agreed to conduct hypnosis sessions over FaceTime because she lived far from where I was based.

She booked an appointment, but according to her, she was fearful it would end up being a scam. Her first hour of therapy was like a typical therapy session. We discussed her challenges, feelings, and background.

After these sessions, she realized that she was not aware of her food and body issues. We discovered that a particular aspect of her childhood was the root cause of her eating disorders. I remember when she learned about it, she became a sobbing mess!

We established that her food issues were directly correlated to the traumatic events that happened during her childhood. We spent little time on it. We moved on to discuss Trina's daily routines, which mainly consisted of distractions from her hunger through work, social life, and sleep.

I introduced her to a new routine that required her to eat small meals throughout the day. However, Trina revealed that she didn't know how to eat without stopping. But I reminded her that she knows how and all she needed to do was to take control.

We did a hypnosis session where I took Trina back to the first time she started feeling inferior and ugly. I helped her into an encounter with the young her and corrected the mess that had started years ago. I told her in her hypnosis state to use positive affirmations on the younger version of herself.

After the session was over, she stated how free she was feeling. We did the same for two other memories, and Trina was no longer feeling "heavily burdened."

We then came back to her present life, where we thoroughly went through her daily routine. I made her confess how she was in control of everything, including every meal, snack and that she could stop when full. I also encouraged her to congratulate herself for being in control of her life and decision.

Trina states that even though her priority was to lose weight, our sessions together helped her change her perspective. She discovered that her weight was not the problem. However, multiple years of yo-yo dieting, binging, starvation, and punishing herself were hurting her mental and physical health.

She needed a sustainable, healthy change to enjoy a longer and happier life. She needed to take a trip to her subconscious mind and deal with the nasty thoughts and feelings she had internalized over the years. I am glad we found a lasting solution to her issues.

Trina's story summarizes what this book is all about – finding a healthier and more sustainable lifestyle without punishing yourself. You see, the same way you subconsciously gain weight is the same way you will lose it. Luckily, hypnotherapy does not put pressure on you to lose weight. Instead, it encourages you to look inside and discover the best version of yourself. After doing this, weight loss just comes as a bonus. Amazing! Right?

I understand that there are many ideas about hypnotherapy, and that is why the first chapter begins by clearing the air on what it is. I have also explained to you how self-hypnosis for weight loss is performed.

In the second section of the book, I have covered in-depth several methods you can use in your weight loss journey, including Gastric Band Hypnotherapy for Weight Loss, Meditation, Positive Affirmations, and how to create habits for weight loss. I have also created an entire chapter that will help you understand how you can stay motivated in your weight loss journey.

The third part of the book covers critical aspects of weight loss that many people have misunderstood for a long time. I have elaborated the principles of dieting and eating and the principles of nutrition. All these principles also encourage you to go easy on yourself and avoid denying your body essential nutrients.

Another key thing that affects your weight loss journey is how you track progress. I have given you the right tactics you can use to ensure you don't focus on the wrong things to put unnecessary pressure on yourself.

So, are you having trouble losing weight? Have you found out what you ought to do to embark on a sustainable weight loss journey? Start by joining my exclusive community for more relatable content and a FREE BONUS book: Weight Loss 101 – Key Factors for Weight Loss Success.

What are you waiting for? Now is the time to act!

A SHORT MESSAGE FROM THE AUTHOR

Hey, are you enjoying the book? I'd love to hear your thoughts!

Many readers do not know how hard reviews are to come by, and how much they help an author.

I would be incredibly grateful if you could take just 60 seconds to write a brief review on Amazon, even if it's just a few sentences!

Thank you for taking the time to share your thoughts!

Your review will genuinely make a difference for me and help gain exposure for my work.

J. W. Chloe

REFERENCES

American Board of Neuro Linguistics Programming. (2017). *Hypnotic Induction Techniques.* https://www.abh-abnlp.com/hypnotic-induction-techniques/

Adejuwon, S. (2018). *Ten Habits of People Who Lose Weight and Keep it off.* The Conversation. https://theconversation.com/ten-habits-of-people-who-lose-weight-and-keep-it-off-101387

Adele, H. (2021). *Setting Realistic Expectations For Weight Loss.* DietDoctor. https://www.dietdoctor.com/weight loss/realistic-expectations

Amy, R. (2020). *52 Weight Loss Affirmations To Start Using Today.* Health Beet. https://healthbeet.org/52-weight loss-affirmations-to-start-using-today/

Behavior Modification. (n.d.). Serenity Hypnosis. Retrieved July 19, 2021, from https://serenityhypnosis.com/Modifying-behaviour

Bowers, K. S. (1992). Imagination and Dissociation in Hypnotic Responding. *International Journal of Clinical and Experimental Hypnosis, 40,* 253–275.

Brooks, S. (2020). *31 Hypnosis Techniques.* The British Hypnosis Research & Training Institute. https://britishhypnosisresearch.com/hypnosis-techniques/

Brown, R. J., Oakley, D.A. (2004). *An Integrative Cognitive Theory of Hypnosis and Hypnotizability.* In: M. Heap, R.J. Brown, D.A. Oakley (Eds.), The Highly Hypnotizable Person. New York: Brunner - Routledge.

Caroline, P. (2017). *16 Ways to Motivate Yourself to Lose Weight.* Healthline. https://www.healthline.com/nutrition/weight loss-motivation-tips

Caroline, R. (2020). *15 Affirmations That Helped Me Lose Weight.* Mind Body Green. https://www.mindbodygreen.com/0-8370/15-affirmations-that-will-help-you-lose-weight.html

Crawford, H. J., & Gruzelier, J. . (1992). A Midstream View of the Neuropsychophysiology of Hypnosis: Recent Research

Meagan, D. (2020). *Most Diets Don't Work for Weight Loss After a Year: Here's Why*. Healthline. https://www. healthline.com/health-news/diets-work-for-one-year

Meditation For Weight Loss. (2021). Headspace. Retrieved July 19, 2021, from https://www.headspace.com/ meditation/weight loss

Meg, S. (2010). *Why Diets Don't Work... and What Does*. Psychology Today. https://www.psychologytoday.com/au/ blog/changepower/201010/why-diets-dont-work-and-what-does

Mendel, M. (n.d.). *The Ultimate Guide to Hypnotic Inductions*. Retrieved July 19, 2021, from https:// mikemandelhypnosis.com/hypnosis-training/hypnotic-inductions-ultimate-guide/

Michael, N. (2017). *Natural Eating*. HUFFPOST. https:// www.huffpost.com/entry/natural-eating_b_6692304

Mummy, T. H. (2021). *How To Stay Motivated When Losing Weight*. The Healthy Mummy. https://www. healthymummy.com/how-to-stay-motivated-when-losing-weight/

Nancy, C. (2016). 50 Weight Loss Affirmations. Retrieved from Committed To Myself website: https:// committedtomyself.com/50-weight loss-affirmations/

Positive Affirmations to Help with Weight Loss. (n.d.). Retrieved from DeStress.com website: https://www.destress.com/relaxation-techniques/positive-affirmations/positive-affirmations-to-help-with-weight loss/

Psychology, B. (n.d.). Altered States of Consciousness. Retrieved from Lumen website: https://courses.lumenlearning.com/boundless-psychology/chapter/altered-states-of-consciousness/

Rachael, L. (2018). 10 Morning Habits That Help You Lose Weight. Retrieved from Healthline website: https://www.healthline.com/nutrition/weight loss-morning-habits

Revenga Juan. (2016). 4 Golden Rules to Eat Well. Retrieved from PATIA website: https://www.patiadiabetes.com/en/golden-rules-to-eat-healthy/

Robert, B. (2017). The Psychology of Weight Loss: Managing Expectations. Retrieved from RdB Nutrition website: https://www.robertbarrington.net/the-psychology-of-weight loss-managing-expectations/

Robert, S. (2020). When Dieting Doesn't Work. Retrieved from Harvard Health Publishing website: https://www.health.harvard.edu/blog/when-dieting-doesnt-work-2020052519889

Sadhguru. (2013). How To Eat Properly - 5 Tips For Healthy Eating. Retrieved from Isha Institute of Inner Sciences website: https://isha.sadhguru.org/ca/en/wisdom/article/how-to-eat-properly?
gclid=Cj0KCQjwytOEBhD5ARIsANnRjVj4aKBXRUf7aT7
KlG2tKayoX2Ac_RUmCrHSQk7KusHfvrn_O3C49dcaAndq
EALw_wcB

Scott, H. (2005). Ten Golden Rules of Dieting. Retrieved from Wightloss.com.au website: http://www.weightloss.com.au/diet/diet-articles/golden-rules-of-dieting.html

Sheila, G. (2019). Gastric Band Weight Loss. Retrieved from Hypfocus website: https://www.hypfocus.com.au/virtual-gastric band-melbourne-weight loss-hypnotherapy.html

Simone, A. (2021). Fad Diets. Retrieved from Sports Dietitians Australia website: https://www.sportsdietitians.com.au/fad-diets/

Simple Habits to Lose Weight Without Trying So Hard, Backed by Science. (2020). Retrieved from Eat This, Not That website: https://www.eatthis.com/simple-weight loss-habits/

Spanos, N.P. (1986). Hypnotic Behavior: A Social Psychological Interpretation of Amnesia, Analgesia, and "Trance Logic." *Behavioral and Brain Sciences, 9,* 449-502.

Steve, K. (2020). Taking Body Measurements: The Ultimate Guide For Tracking Fitness. Retrieved from NerdFitness website: https://www.nerdfitness.com/blog/how-to-track-progress/

Teamvida. (2020). Extrinsic vs Intrinsic Motivation. Retrieved from VIDA website: https://vidafitness.com.au/extrinsic-and-intrinsic-motivation/

Terence, W. (2021). The Subconscious Mind and Hypnosis. Retrieved from Self Hypnosis website: https://www.selfhypnosis.com/the-subconscious-mind/

Tom, H. (2021). How Hypnosis Works. Retrieved from How Stuff Works website: https://science.howstuffworks.com/science-vs-myth/extrasensory-perceptions/hypnosis2.htm

Valerie, G. (2015). Hypnosis For Behavior Change. Retrieved from The Flow Center website: https://theflowcenter.com/hypnosis-for-behavior-change/

Wiktoria, B. (2021). The Top 10 Ways To Track Fitness Progress Like A Pro. Retrieved from SHAPE website: https://www.shapescale.com/blog/tracking/how-to-track-fitness-progress/

Woody, E., Bowers, K. (1994). A Frontal Assault on Dissociated Control. In: Lynn, S.J., Rhue, J.W. (Eds.), Dissociation:

Jessica, S. (2020). *The 23 Best Weight loss Motivation Tips.* SHAPE. https://www.shape.com/weight loss/tips-plans/22-ways-stay-motivated-lose-weight

Kate, B. (2017). *Hypnosis and Weight Loss.* Choice. https://www.choice.com.au/health-and-body/diet-and-fitness/weight loss/articles/hypnosis-and-weight loss

Kathleen, Z. (2021). *Top 10 Habits That Can Help You Lose Weight.* Nourish. https://www.webmd.com/diet/obesity/features/top-10-habits-that-can-help-you-lose-weight#1

Kihlstrom, J.F. (1985). Hypnosis. *Annual Review of Psychology*, 36, 385 - 418.

Kirsch, I. (1985). Response Expectancy as a Determinant of Experience and Behavior. *Annual Review of Psychology*, 40, 1189–1202. Retrieved from http://www.jgh.ca/uploads/Psychiatry/Links/kirsch_1985.pdf

Kirsch, I., & Lynn, S. . (1997). Hypnotic Involuntaries and The Automaticity of Everyday Life. *American Journal of Clinical Hypnosis, 40,* 329–348.

Kris, G. (2020). *How To Lose Weight Fast: 3 Simple Steps, Based on Science.* Healthline. https://www.healthline.com/nutrition/how-to-lose-weight-as-fast-as-possible

Krissy, B. (2017). *What To Do If You Want To Lose Weight - But Just Can't Motivate Yourself To Get Started.* Women's Health. https://www.womenshealthmag.com/weight loss/a19951279/how-to-get-motivated-to-lose-weight/

Linnea, Z. (2020). *Can Meditation Help You Lose Weight?* Woman's World. https://www.womansworld.com/posts/health/everything-you-need-to-know-about-meditation-and-weight loss-120305

Lisa, W. (2021). *7 Positive Affirmations to Improve Your Well-Being.* Healthline. https://www.healthline.com/nutrition/affirmations-for-weight loss

Malia, F. (2020). *How To Find Motivation to Lose Weight.* VeryWell Fit. https://www.verywellfit.com/how-to-motivate-yourself-to-lose-weight-3496383

Marisa, P. (2019). *The Difference Between Your Conscious and Subconscious Mind.* https://marisapeer.com/the-differences-between-your-conscious-and-subconscious-mind/

Maureen, M. (2020). *Why Diets Don't Work.* Nutritionist Resource. https://www.nutritionist-resource.org.uk/blog/2020/10/02/why-diets-dont-work

Clinical and Theoretical Perspectives. Guilford Press, New York, USA, pp.52-79.

Zahra, B. (2016). 14 Small Lifestyle Habits That Will Help You Lose Weight. Retrieved from SELF website: https://www.self.com/story/small-lifestyle-habits-help-lose-weight

Made in the USA
Monee, IL
24 November 2021

and Future Directions. *Contemporary Hypnosis Research*, 227–266.

Dale, P. (n.d.). *Four Golden Rules Of Healthy Eating For Life*. Women's Transformation Studio. Retrieved July 19, 2021, from https://www.womenstransformationstudio.com.au/the-four-golden-rules-of-healthy-eating-for-life/

Diane, P. (2012). *Use Affirmations For Weight Loss Success*. https://dianepetrella.com/blog/affirmations/use-affirmations-for-weight loss-success/

Dienes, Z., & Perner, J. (2007). The Cold Control Theory of Hypnosis. In G. Jamieson (Ed.), Hypnosis and Conscious States: The Cognitive Neuroscience Perspective. Oxford University Press, pp 293-314.

Dr. Whalley, M. (n.d.). *Scientific Theories of Hypnosis*. Hypnosis and Suggestion. Retrieved July 19, 2021, from https://hypnosisandsuggestion.org/theories-of-hypnosis.html

Dr. Whalley, M. (n.d.). *Theories of Hypnosis*. Dr. Goodman. http://drdgoodman.com/wp-content/uploads/2016/02/theories_of_hypnosis1.pdf

Elman, D. (2019). *Hypnosis Inductions*. Hypnosis 101. https://www.hypnosis101.com/hypnosis/hypnosis-inductions/

Gastric Band Hypnosis. (2021). Hypnotherapy Directory. Retrieved July 19, 2021, from https://www.hypnotherapy-directory.org.uk/articles/gastric band.html

Gillian, H. (2017). *Can Hypnotherapy Help You Lose Weight.* Patient. https://patient.info/news-and-features/can-hypnotherapy-help-you-lose-weight

Hilgard, E. R., Crawford, H. J., & Wert, A. (1979). The Stanford Hypnotic Arm Levitation Induction and Test (SHALT): A Six Minute Induction and Measurement Scale. *Psychological Review, 27*(2), 111–124.

Hypnosis, N. (n.d.). *An Explanation of the Most Common Hypnotic Induction Techniques.* Natural Hypnosis. https://www.naturalhypnosis.com/blog/hypnotic-induction-techniques

Jan, D. P. (2021). *Hypnosis and the Power of the Subconscious Mind.* M1 Psychology. https://m1psychology.com/hypnosis-and-the-power-of-the-subconscious-mind/

Jenn, H. (2014). *Does Meditation Help You Lose Weight.* WebMD website. https://www.webmd.com/balance/features/meditation-hypertension-and-weight loss

Jennifer, S. (2021). *How to Stay Motivated During Weight Loss.* VeryWell Fit. https://www.verywellfit.com/stay-motivated-3496369